UROLOGICAL
DISORDERS OF THE
DOG AND CAT

INVESTIGATION, DIAGNOSIS AND TREATMENT

Peter E Holt

BVMS, PhD, DipECVS, CBiol, FIBiol, FHEA, FRCVS

Professor of Veterinary Surgery
School of Clinical Veterinary Science
University of Bristol
Langford, Bristol, UK

T0132740

MANSON PUBLISHING/THE VETERINARY PRESS

This book is dedicted to: the memory of my father Eric R Holt whose enthusiasm for my work was, and still is, a constant source of encouragement to me; my Mum for allowing her first born the chance to stay on at school and go to University, contrary to family tradition; my wife, Sylvia, my best friend, supporter and, when required, critic; my sons, Brandon and Andrew, who would probably have liked to have seen more of their Dad as children and of whom I am immensely proud; Alan Case, who got me through A-level Physics but then died too young; John Lamb (drummer *extraordinaire*), 'Cappy' Powell and an anonymous newsagent who helped teach me about selflessness, values and compassion; and my mentors Sir William Weipers, Professor Donald Lawson, Professor Jimmy Campbell, Professor Harold Pearson and Dr Christine Gibbs.

Softcover edition 2011

Copyright © 2008 Manson Publishing Ltd

ISBN: 978-1-84076-176-4

A CIP catalogue record for this book is available from the British Library.

For full details of all Manson Publishing Ltd titles please write to:
Manson Publishing Ltd, 73 Corringham Road, London NW11 7DL, UK.
Tel: +44(0)20 8905 5150
Fax: +44(0)20 8201 9233
Email: manson@mansonpublishing.com
Website: www.mansonpublishing.com

Commissioning editor: Jill Northcott
Project manager: Ayala Kingsley
Copy editor: Peter Beynon
Cover and book design: Ayala Kingsley
Layout and illustration: DiacriTech, Chennai, India
Colour reproduction: Tenon & Polert Colour Scanning Ltd, Hong Kong
Printed by: Grafos SA, Barcelona, Spain

Contents

3

Foreword

Be careful about reading health books. You may die of a misprint.
Mark Twain (1835–1910)

THIS BOOK IS AIMED first and foremost at being a practical guide for the small animal veterinary practitioner. For this reason, the investigative procedures and surgical techniques described are those that the author considers practicable in a reasonably well-equipped veterinary practice. The book is not intended to be read from cover to cover. Apart from certificate or diploma examination candidates, I am aware of few people who do this. Rather, this book is meant to be referred to for practical information on a specific problem as and when the need arises, and copious cross-referencing is used to direct the reader to related material within the book. I have always investigated as well as treated my own cases and no apology is made for allocating a large section of this book to the investigation of animals with urological signs. An accurate diagnosis is the foundation upon which any treatment plan is built. Detailed descriptions of advanced techniques such as scintigraphy and MRI or CT scanning will not be described. Apart from the lack of facilities in most practices, these are specialized techniques requiring specialized equipment and expertise in their use and interpretation.

Mark Twain, if he was alive, would be reassured by the professional assistance I have had in the production of this book and I am grateful to the following for their help and support:

- Dr Frances Barr for assistance with ultrasonographic illustrations (figures 85, 259–262) and advice.
- Dr Kostas Papasouliotis for advice on normal laboratory values.
- Mr A Skuse for advice on the staining of cytological specimens.
- The late, great Professor Harold Pearson for permission to use figures 432, 433.
- Mr Alasdair Hotston Moore for permission to use figures 365–367.
- Dr Dick White and Mr Jonathan Bray for allowing me to use their figures as a basis for figures 313–317.
- My surgical colleagues and clinical scholars at Langford for keeping me on my toes, especially Mr Hotston Moore, Dr Martin Owen, Dr Eithne Comerford and Mr Christopher Shales.
- Mr John Conibear, Mr Malcolm Parsons and Ms Tracey Dewey who took most of the photographs used in this book.
- The anaesthetists and veterinary nurses who helped in the management of the cases used to illustrate this book.
- The students who helped to care for many of these animals.
- Special thanks to Professor Elizabeth Stone and Mr Rob White, who reviewed the draft of this book for the publishers, for their constructive comments.

The evidence base in many areas of veterinary urology is thin and, sometimes, controversial (e.g. the necessity to ligate the renal artery and vein separately or not during nephrectomy). This book is therefore based almost entirely upon my own experiences, good and bad, and I would commend to the reader the following quotation by Carolyn Coats (1988) in her book 'Things Your Dad Always Told You But You Didn't Want To Hear':

Learn from the mistakes of others; you may not live long enough to make them all yourself.

Abbreviations

CT	computed tomography
DHTest	dihydrotestosterone
DNA	deoxyribonucleic acid
ECG	electrocardiogram
FLUTD	feline lower urinary tract disease
FSH	follicle stimulating hormone
FUS	feline urological syndrome
IVU	intravenous urography
LH	luteinizing hormone
LHRH	luteinizing hormone releasing hormone
LMN	lower motor neurone
MCH	mean corpuscular haemoglobin
MCHC	mean corpuscular haemoglobin concentration
MCV	mean corpuscular volume
MRI	magnetic resonance imaging
ND:YAG	neodymium: yttrium aluminium garnet (laser)
NSAID	non-steroidal anti-inflammatory drug
PCV	packed cell volume
RBC	red blood cell(s)
RNA	ribonucleic acid
Test	testosterone
UMN	upper motor neurone
WBC	white blood cell(s)

INVESTIGATION OF ANIMALS WITH UROLOGICAL SIGNS

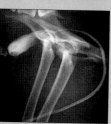

1 Clinical assessment

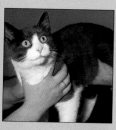

2 Radiographic investigations

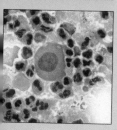

3 Other diagnostic aids

1 Clinical assessment

But most physical defensive reactions are of the same scarcely recognisable and, so to speak, indirect nature, and their purposeful character also has only been recognised through deep investigation and exact observation.

Carl Jung (1875–1961)

IN THIS CHAPTER, a brief account is given of the clinical assessment of small animals presented with signs of urological disease.

Most animals with urological presenting signs can be divided into those presenting primarily with dysuria, haematuria, urinary incontinence or frequency/urgency. The main conditions leading to these signs are listed in *Tables 1–5*. Some sex predispositions are obvious (e.g. prostatic disease), but symbols based on the author's experiences appear alongside conditions potentially responsible for the urological signs; m = commoner in male animals; f = commoner in female animals; n = no apparent sex predisposition.

Table 1 **Dysuria**

Urethral prolapse (m)

Prostatic disorders (m)

Bladder neck neoplasia (f)

Urethral neoplasia (f)

Urethral trauma (n)

Urethritis (f)

Urethral stricture (n)

Neurogenic dysuria (n)

Bladder displacement/entrapment (m)

Functional disorders (e.g. dyssynergia [m], bladder atony [m])

External resistance to urine outflow (e.g. ureterocoele [rarely] [n])

Table 2 **Haematuria**

Urinary tract infection (n)

Urolithiasis (n)

Prostatic disorders (m)

Urinary tract neoplasia (n)

Urinary tract trauma (n)

Idiopathic renal haemorrhage (n)

Urethral prolapse (m)

Table 3 **Congenital urinary incontinence**

Ureteral ectopia (f)

Congenital urethral sphincter mechanism incompetence (f)

Bladder hypoplasia (n)

Pervious urachus (n)

Intersexuality (n)

Congenital neurological abnormalities (n)

Table 4 **Acquired urinary incontinence**

Acquired urethral sphincter mechanism incompetence (f)

Prostatic disorders (m)

Bladder/urethral neoplasia (f)

Uretero- or vesicovaginal fistula (f)

Acquired neurological conditions (n)

Overflow incontinence with chronic retention (m)

Detrusor overactivity/hyperactivity/instability (n)

Table 5 **Frequency/urgency** (pollakiuria)

Cystitis/urethritis (f)

Cystolithiasis (f)

Bladder/urethral neoplasia (f)

Prostatic disease (m)

Bladder hypoplasia/detrusor overactivity/hyperactivity/instability (n)

Lower urinary tract trauma (n)

The clinical assessment of animals with these signs can be divided into history taking (**1**) and clinical examination (**2–15**) for the purposes of description, but these two activities are closely interrelated; further questioning of the owner may be suggested by clinical findings, whilst the history may point to a particular type of examination.

1 A good history is essential. In many animals with urological signs, especially incontinent dogs and cats, there may be few or no detectable abnormalities on clinical examination, but a good history will usually suggest which part of the urinary tract merits more detailed ancillary investigations. As well as the breed, sex and age of the animal, the presence or absence and, where relevant, frequency and severity of the following should be determined:

- Entire or neutered animal.
- Anorexia/inappetence.
- Polydipsia/polyuria.
- Dysuria. Differentiate straining to pass urine in obstructed animals from faecal tenesmus or urinary tenesmus with the bladder small or empty.
- Anuria.
- Oliguria.
- Nocturia.
- Urinary incontinence. Differentiate from inappropiate micturition (e.g. behavioural or the untrained puppy).
- Urinary frequency/urgency (pollakiuria).
- Haematuria. Differentiate from haemoglobinuria and determine the phase of urination during which most blood is present; for example, in male dogs with prostatic disease the first part of the stream may be most bloody, bladder urothelial tumours often bleed towards the end of micturition and the urine is usually equally bloody throughout micturition in cases of renal haemorrhage. However, these are not hard and fast rules.

- Pyuria. Determine if a purulent urethral discharge is also present (e.g. the dog with prostatic abscessation).
- Urethral discharge. Differentiate from preputial or vaginal discharge and urinary incontinence: determine nature of discharge.
- Oversexuality (in males).
- Vulval/preputial licking.
- Neurological signs.

2 A detailed clinical examination in animals with obstructive dysuria is less of a priority than relief of the dysuria. Prolonged bladder distension may result in bladder wall ischaemia. Initially, this affects the urothelium, which may become necrotic and slough, as illustrated in this dog five days after acute dysuria. Sloughed urothelium may be a further cause of obstructive dysuria. If acute bladder distension is prolonged, the ischaemia may involve all layers of the bladder wall and the result may be a bladder that is a non-functional, fibrotic sac. In addition, bladder nerve stretching, demyelination and breakdown of tight junctions may occur, resulting in neurogenic dysuria following relief of the obstruction. Dysuria should be relieved by catheterization or cystocentesis (see Chapter 3, Centesis).

3 Urinary incontinence. A continuous dripping incontinence in a juvenile animal may suggest ureteral ectopia, which was present in this Golden Retriever, but it can also be associated with uretero- or vesico-vaginal fistula and paradoxical overflow incontinence associated with obstructive or neurogenic dysuria.

4 Intermittent, more copious incontinence, which occurs predominantly during recumbency, is suggestive of urethral sphincter mechanism incompetence. These signs are not pathognomonic and clinical, contrast radiographic and laboratory examinations are required to make an accurate diagnosis.

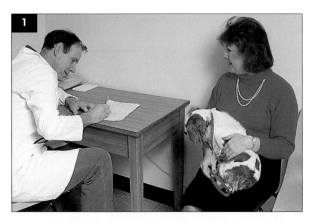

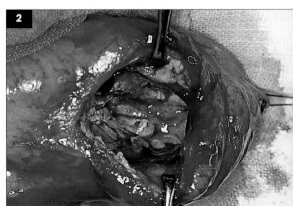

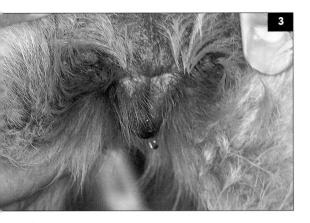

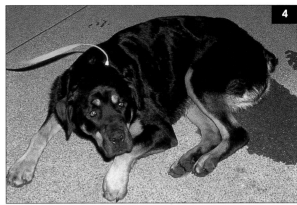

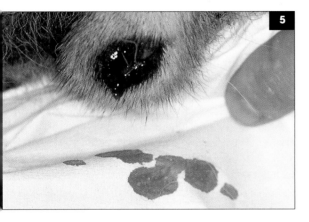

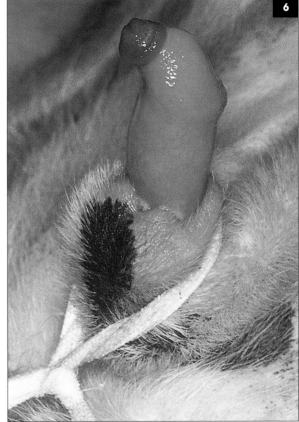

5 A bloody urethral discharge in male dogs is sometimes mistaken by the owners for haematuria or incontinence of bloody urine. A good history should differentiate these and clinical examination will exclude lesions of the prepuce and/or penis as the source of haemorrhage. If the urine is said to be clear of or to contain much less blood, such a discharge suggests a prostatic or urethral disorder. Bleeding in this dog originated from the prostate gland.

6 A bloody preputial discharge may be due to a preputial or penile lesion. In the case of this Bulldog, a urethral prolapse was the source of the haemorrhage.

7 Clinical examination revealed that the purulent discharge in this dog was urethral rather than preputial in origin. Cytological and bacteriological examinations of the discharge should be performed to confirm its nature, obtain antibiotic sensitivities and look for the presence of malignant cells. This Boxer had a prostatic abscess.

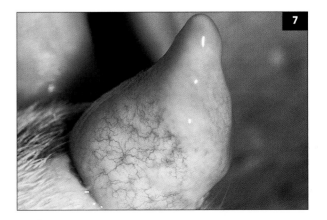

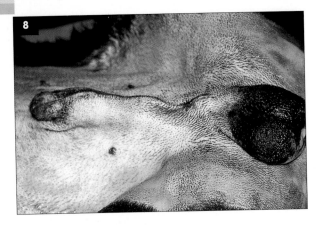

8 The urethra should be palpated for abnormal masses. This dysuric German Shepherd Dog has a firm mass at the caudal end of the os penis (just cranial to the scrotum). Masses in this region may be large urethral calculi, but these are not always palpable. This dog has a tumour of the os penis (a chondrosarcoma). Its treatment is illustrated later (see **187–199**).
The pelvic urethra can be palpated *per rectum* in males and females and examination of the female urethra can be performed *per vaginam* in large bitches. In male and female cats, external and rectal palpations only are practicable, although rectal examination of this species usually requires sedation or general anaesthesia.

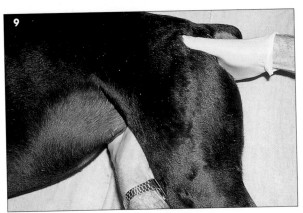

9 In male dogs the prostate is best examined by a combination of abdominal and rectal palpations. In the case of a right-handed person, the left hand is used to push the prostate caudodorsally onto the finger of the right hand, which is in the rectum. If the animal is recumbent, palpation is easier in right lateral recumbency (as shown) for a right handed person. Left-handed clinicians should reverse this advice. The prostate is examined for size, symmetry, texture and pain; the value of the findings in differential diagnosis is summarized in *Table 11* (p. 91).

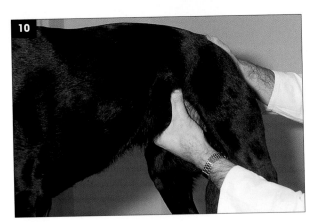

10, 11 Bladder palpation is best performed with one hand (unless the size of the animal or bladder makes this impossible) (**10**). The size, degree of turgidity and thickness of the bladder wall and the presence of abnormal masses should be determined. The detection of crepitation suggests the presence of multiple cystoliths or bladder wall mineralization. Bladder wall thickness can be assessed (as long as the bladder is not distended with urine) between the thumb and fingers as the (doubled) bladder wall is pinched between them (**11**) .

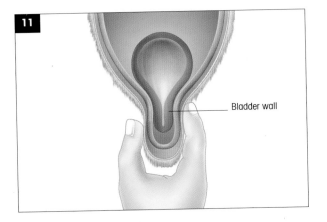

Bladder wall

12 The kidneys can be palpated in the craniodorsal part of the abdomen. If the animal is sufficiently relaxed, it is possible to palpate deep to the costal arch, as illustrated. This may be necessary to locate the right kidney which is more cranial than the left.

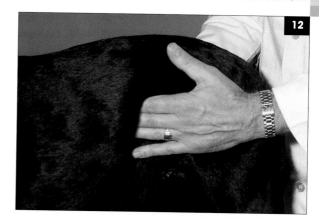

13 The kidneys of cats are more easily located than those of dogs and, in cats and small dogs, may be palpated using one hand. The kidney position, size, texture and shape should be assessed. In the author's experience, renal pain is difficult to assess in small animals. Dogs and cats with renal lesions that one would expect to be painful frequently show no signs of pain, while spinal pain in animals is sometimes misdiagnosed as renal pain.

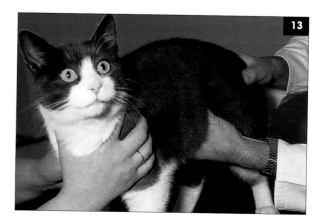

14 Micturition and urinary continence control depend upon complex neuromuscular activity and coordination. During micturition the impulse of the pelvic nerve causes contraction (+); that of the pudendal and hypogastric nerves causes relaxation (−). Most clinicians are familiar with the animal with thoracolumbar spinal disease that develops urinary retention as part of a more widespread problem, but neurogenic urological problems can occur without overt neurological limb abnormalities. This is particularly true if the sacral segments of the spinal cord or their nerve roots are affected. If so, much of the nerve supply to hindlimb musculature may be intact (since it originates from caudal lumbar spinal cord segments and is cranial to the lesion) and the animal may show little, if any, hindlimb gait abnormalities. However, evidence of cauda equina disease may be detectable (i.e. bladder and possibly rectal paralysis, tail paresis or paralysis and perineal skin desensitization).

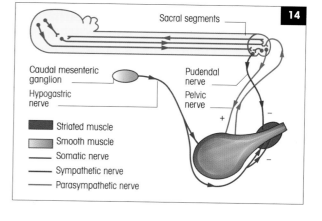

15 A blackboard or wipe-clean board is a useful addition to the consulting room. It greatly facilitates explanations of possible diagnoses, further investigative procedures, potential treatments and complications to the owner of the animal.

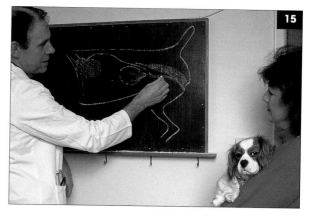

2 Radiographic investigations

Isn't life a series of images that change as they repeat themselves?
Andy Warhol (1928–1987)

RADIOGRAPHIC INVESTIGATIONS are frequently required in the differential diagnosis of conditions leading to urological presenting signs in small animals. Plain abdominal radiographs are mandatory and thoracic radiography should not be neglected in cases of suspected malignancy (to examine for the presence of pulmonary metastases). In the majority of cases, plain radiographs alone are insufficient for diagnostic purposes and contrast radiographs are required.

In this chapter, intravenous urography, vagino-urethrography, urethrography and cystography will be described. These are the commonest techniques employed in urological cases and they are applicable in general practice. The descriptions will concentrate on indications, techniques and problems in technique and interpretation and how to avoid them. No detail of radiographic exposure will be given, since these will vary considerably depending on the equipment available to the reader. In addition, a level of radiographic competence by the reader is assumed.

It is vital that all radiographs are taken when the animal is still. This is particularly important when examining the kidneys, which move caudally and cranially during inspiration and expiration, respectively, due to diaphragmatic movements. Radiographic exposures should, therefore, be made immediately after expiration, during the respiratory pause when the animal is not moving. The exception is thoracic radiography, which is usually performed at full inspiration.

Plain films

Indications
- Urolithiasis (**16–18**).
- Determination of organ size, shape and position (**19**).
- Evidence of local or distant tumour metastases (**20–23**).
- As control films, prior to contrast radiography.

16 Bladder calculi can usually be seen on plain films. Radiographs should be made before the bladder is emptied, as the calculi show up better in a full, rather than an empty, bladder. Non-radiopaque calculi can be demonstrated by double contrast cystography but, somewhat surprisingly, they are not well-outlined by pneumocystography alone. If plain radiographs are not made before positive contrast radiographic techniques, vesical calculi may be obscured by the contrast medium and remain undetected.

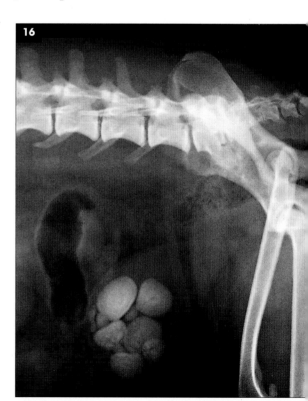

16

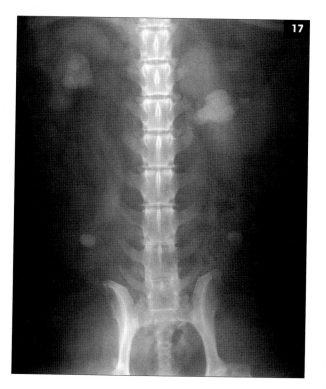

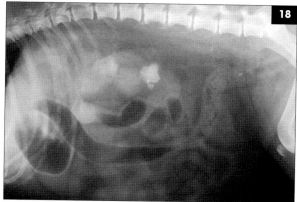

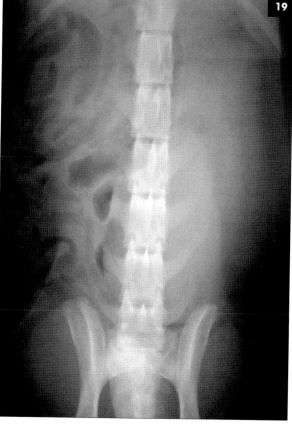

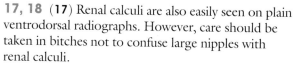

17, 18 (**17**) Renal calculi are also easily seen on plain ventrodorsal radiographs. However, care should be taken in bitches not to confuse large nipples with renal calculi.
(**18**) Lateral abdominal radiography will distinguish between large nipples and renal calculi; the nipples will now be on the ventral abdominal wall, whereas the calculus or calculi will still be in the region of the renal pelvis/pelves in the craniodorsal abdomen.

19 The size, shape and position of urinary tract organs can sometimes be seen on plain films. In many cases, however, contrast radiographic techniques are required more accurately to distinguish urinary tract organs from surrounding soft tissues. In addition, although this dog appears to have an enlarged left kidney on this plain ventrodorsal abdominal radiograph, additional techniques (intravenous urography, ultrasonography, urine laboratory examinations) are required before the reason for the enlargement can be determined (see **32, 33**).

20 Thoracic radiography should always be performed in cases of possible urinary tract malignancy. This aged Poodle was treated by castration and oestrogens for 12 months for benign prostatic enlargement. On presentation, the dog screamed during any attempt to examine or handle it. The reason for the pain is apparent in the next two illustrations, but a simple thoracic radiograph would have demonstrated that this was not a benign condition.

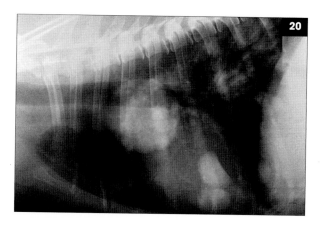

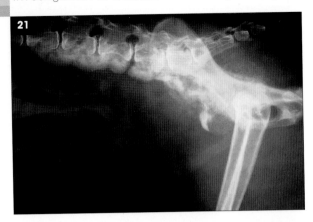

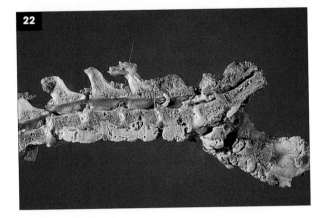

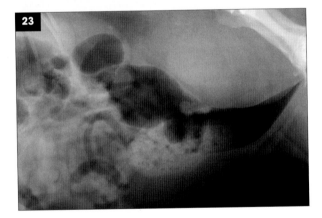

21, 22 (**21**) A plain lateral caudal abdominal radiograph of the dog in **20**. The periosteal bone reactions on the pelvis and sublumbar/sacral vertebrae are highly suggestive of intrapelvic malignancy (in this case, prostatic carcinoma), but are frequently not neoplastic themselves.
(**22**) Postmortem specimen from the dog in **20** and **21**. The periosteal bone reactions can be seen. A metastasis from the prostatic carcinoma is present in the body of the 6th lumbar vertebra.

23 In cases of suspected malignancy, the soft tissues ventral to the caudal lumbar and sacral vertebrae should be examined for evidence of sublumbar/iliac lymph node enlargement, suggesting lymphatic spread. Ultrasonography is a more sensitive method of detecting subtle enlargement. In some instances the enlargement of the sublumbar lymph nodes may be responsible for the urological signs. Dysuria and dyschezia in this dog are due to external pressure on the bladder neck/proximal urethra and rectum by a neoplastic sublumbar lymph node (lymphosarcoma).

Techniques

THE POSITIONING TECHNIQUES for radiography of urinary tract organs are illustrated in the sections on contrast radiographic procedures (see **36–44**). Thoracic and distal male canine urethral radiography are illustrated below (**24–26**).

24, 25 Thoracic radiographs should be made at full inspiration, as this improves the radiographic contrast between pulmonary masses and surrounding air. In anaesthetized animals, this is achieved by forcibly inflating the lungs via the endotracheal tube.
(**24**) For ventrodorsal radiography, the animal is supported in a sponge (or other radiolucent) cradle. The forelimbs are extended using sandbags and the X-ray beam is centred midway along the sternum.
(**25**) During lateral thoracic radiography, the forelimbs are again extended and the sternum is elevated to the level of the vertebral column with a radiolucent wedge. The X-ray beam is centred at the levels of the caudal edge of the scapula and just over a third of the way up the thoracic wall from the sternum. Right and left lateral thoracic radiographs are usually performed for the diagnosis of pulmonary metastases.

26 The penile and ischial urethra in the male dog is best radiographed with the hindlimbs flexed cranially using sandbags and the X-ray beam centred on the penile/ischial urethra. In this way the stifle joints and/or femurs are not superimposed on the caudal penile urethra (see also **29, 30**).

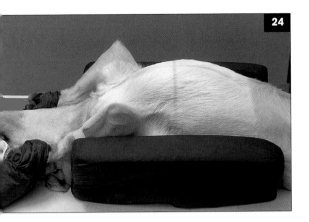

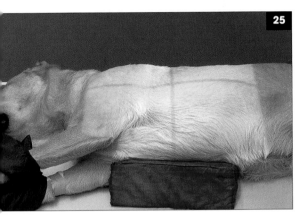

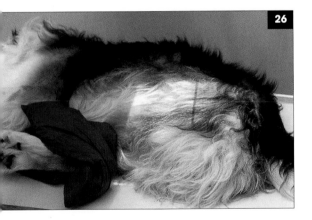

Problems

MANY PROBLEMS are due to incorrect radiographic exposure or positioning. The latter is described below and time spent on obtaining correct exposures is never wasted. Other problems are associated with the presence of overlying viscera or abnormal, but clinically insignificant, tissues (**27–30**).

27 Care should be taken in interpretation when other viscera overlie urinary tract organs. The problem of nipples being misdiagnosed as renal calculi has already been mentioned (**17, 18**). In this illustration, mineralized material in overlying bowel may be confused with vesical calculi; a radiograph made in the other plane (in this case, a ventrodorsal radiograph) would clarify the situation.

28 Bony reactions or separate centres of ossification of the caudal os penis may be mistaken for urethral calculi in dysuric animals, but they are of no clinical significance (see also Urethral catheterization, p.38). In fact, they are dorsal to the urethra itself and, in case of doubt, this will be apparent if a retrograde positive contrast urethrogram is performed.

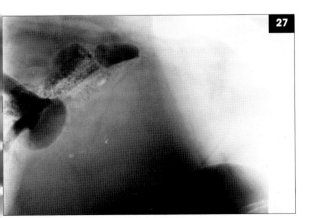

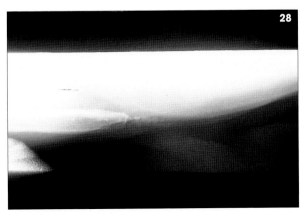

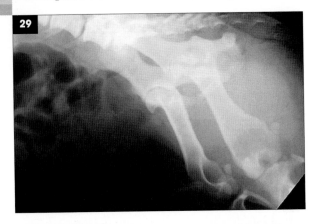

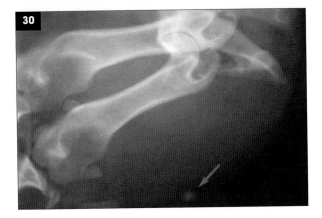

Intravenous urography

Indications
- Urinary incontinence.
- Suspected renal or ureteral lesions.
- Suspected lesions of the bladder trigone.
- An abdominal mass in an otherwise healthy animal.

Some indications for the use of intravenous urography (IVU) are illustrated (**31–35**).

31 IVU is very useful in cases of urinary incontinence. In this example, a dilated ectopic ureter is demonstrated terminating beyond the bladder neck. (NB: Retrograde contrast techniques are frequently required to identify the exact site of the ectopic opening.)

32, 33 (**32**) Gross renal lesions are usually demonstrated by IVU. Hydronephrosis may result in bizarre radiographs, as illustrated in this juvenile male Golden Retriever with ureteral ectopia, hydroureter and hydronephrosis (this is the same dog as shown in **19**). (**33**) The reason for the bizarre appearance can be seen in this specimen of the excised kidney and ureter from the animal in **32**. The contrast medium accumulates in the dependant pockets of the hydronephrotic kidney cavity. It is always a surprise that there is any significant excretion of contrast medium at all in cases such as this in which there is only a thin layer of renal tissue remaining.

34 Ureteral lesions are rare, but rupture of the proximal right ureter following ureterolithiasis is demonstrated by IVU in this Golden Retriever (the radiodensity in the cranial abdomen is barium, administered by mouth to investigate the presenting sign of vomiting in this dog). The bilateral nephroliths and the ureteral calculus responsible for the rupture are now obscured by the contrast medium of the IVU, underlining the need for plain radiographs before administration of contrast medium.

35 IVU may prevent unnecessary surgery. In this German Shepherd Dog a mass was palpated in the caudal abdomen during a routine examination. IVU demonstrates that this is an ectopic kidney (arrow), which is of no clinical significance. Ultrasonography, if available, could also have been used to determine the nature of this mass.

29, 30 (**29**) Urethral calculi proximal to the caudal os penis may be obscured by the stifle joints when the dog is positioned with the hindlimbs extended for caudal abdominal radiography (see **44**). However, this position is useful for demonstrating the vesical calculi that are usually also present.
(**30**) The problems are overcome by repeating the radiograph with the limbs flexed forward and the X-ray beam centred on the ischial and penile urethra (see **26**). This is the same dog as in **129** and the urethral calculus responsible for the dysuria can now be seen.

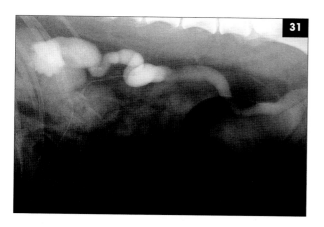

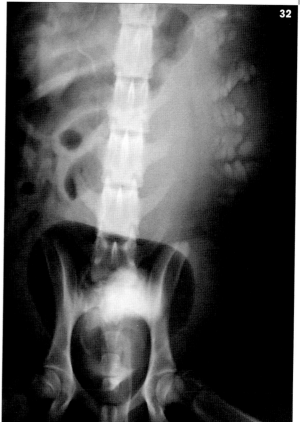

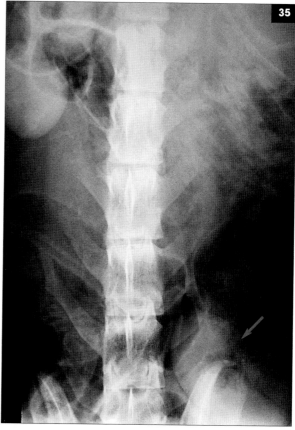

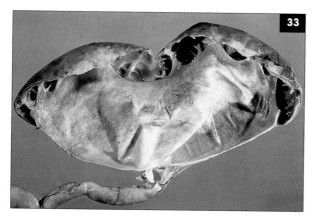

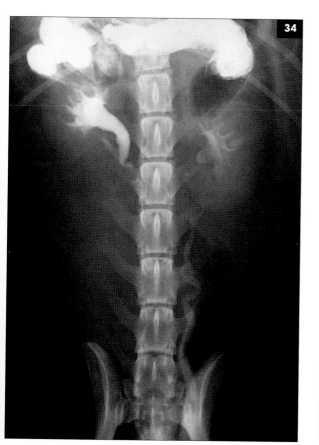

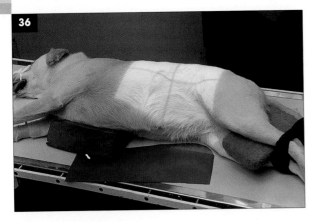

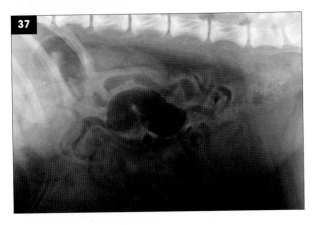

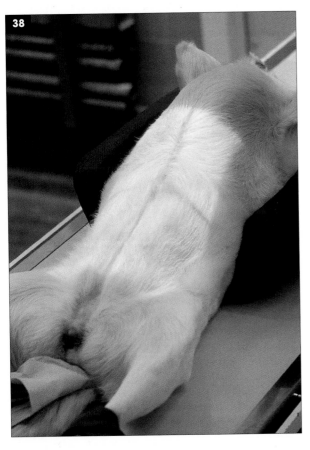

Technique

IT IS IMPORTANT that the gastrointestinal tract is empty, since the presence of ingesta makes radiographic interpretation difficult. This is achieved by the use of enemata. Soapy water enemas are not suitable, as bubbles in the large bowel may be confused with ureters. Proprietary enemas usually work well and the author routinely uses phosphate enemas in medium and large sized dogs and sodium citrate enemas in toy breeds and cats. A third of a phosphate enema is sufficient for a medium-sized dog, half an enema for a large breed and a full enema for giant breeds.

IVU is usually performed under general anaesthesia except in debilitated patients. As with all contrast radiographic techniques, plain radiographs should be made of the area of interest before contrast medium is used. The radiographic timings and positionings illustrated (**36–45**) are for a standard intravenous urogram, but some flexibility is necessary, as dictated by the radiological features that are demonstrated (**46**). The technique is demonstrated in an incontinent (but otherwise normal) bitch, but is identical in cats and in both sexes.

36–45 (**36**) Under general anaesthesia, a plain lateral abdominal radiograph is made centred on the sublumbar region at the level of the umbilicus. Right lateral recumbency is preferred, as this results in better separation of the kidneys than left lateral recumbency due to the relative mobility of the left kidney compared with the right. In addition, it is important to standardize the technique. Note the use of a sponge wedge (blue) to lift the sternum to the same level as the spine and a sponge between the hindlimbs to avoid pelvic tilting. These measures are to ensure that a true lateral radiograph is made. Soft sandbags (green) are used to extend the hindlimbs, and a piece of lead sheet (brown) has been used to absorb X-rays ventral to the abdomen in order to reduce scattered radiation. For caudal abdominal radiography, the film should be centred as shown in **44**.

(**37**) The resultant radiograph is examined for evidence of any abnormalities and can be compared with those obtained after contrast administration. It is also used to determine the efficacy of the enema. In this case, some faecal material remains in the descending colon and rectum and should be removed by lavage with saline.

(**38**) The dog is then placed in dorsal recumbency and a ventrodorsal radiograph made, again centred on the umbilicus. Note the use of a sponge cradle to support the thorax. It is not necessary to support the abdomen, so the possibility of a dirty cradle introducing artefacts on the radiograph is avoided. Soft sandbags are again used to extend the hindlimbs. It is important to prevent spillage of urine onto the X-ray

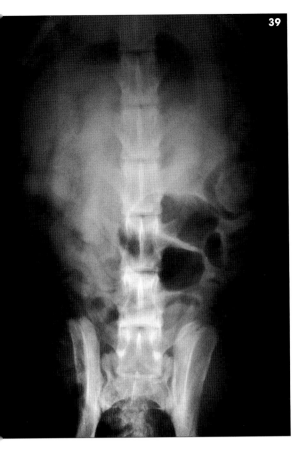

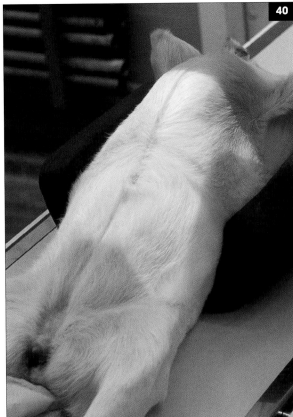

able or/and the animal's coat, particularly after administration of contrast medium. Spilled urine containing contrast medium will show up on subsequent radiographs and may make radiographic interpretation difficult.

(**39**) The radiograph is also examined for evidence of any abnormalities (particularly of the kidneys). The kidneys, particularly the right kidney, are not always visible but, if they are, their position can be assessed and the centring (relative to the umbilicus) adjusted for the next film, the nephrogram.

(**40**) The dog remains in dorsal recumbency and the radiographic beam is centred over the kidneys. If these are not visible on the plain ventrodorsal radiograph, the beam should be centred on a point midway between the umbilicus and the xiphisternum, as illustrated. The bladder is emptied of urine (which is submitted for laboratory examinations) and a small volume of air is introduced into the bladder. It is inadvisable to overdistend the bladder during IVU, as the increased intravesical pressure may compress the intramural part of the ureters, making interpretation of their terminations difficult. One ml of air/kg body weight is usually sufficient. A water-soluble, iodine-based contrast medium containing the equivalent of approximately 400 mg iodine per ml of contrast solution is used in large dogs, while solutions containing about 200 mg iodine per ml are suitable for cats and toy breeds of dog. A bolus of 400 mg/kg of iodine equivalent is administered by rapid intravenous injection. The positioning of the dog is quickly checked (and corrected if the dog has been inadvertently moved during the injection) and the radiograph made immediately. The time is noted, as all further radiographic timings are relative to the time of intravenous injection.

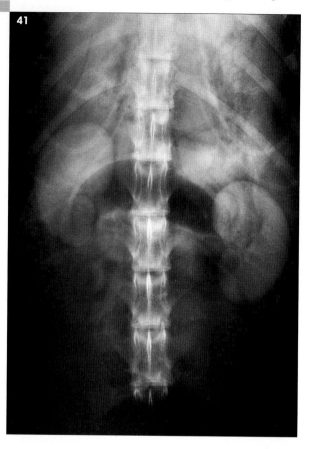

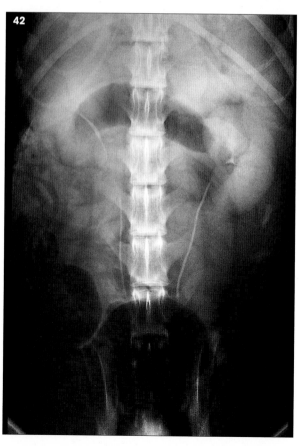

(41) The radiograph made immediately after intravenous injection of contrast medium (the nephogram) should result in good renal opacification. Poor opacification should be interpreted as a sign of possible poor renal function and is an indication for biochemical renal function tests, if these have not already been performed. The nephrogram is examined for number of kidneys, renal position, size and shape, and abnormal filling with contrast medium. If any apparent lucent areas are seen within the kidney(s), the plain radiographs should be examined to ensure that such lucency is not just due to overlying loops of gas-filled bowel.

(42) Five minutes after administration of contrast medium, a ventrodorsal radiograph is made, centred again on the umbilicus. This should show the kidneys, renal pelves and at least the proximal ureters. The renal pelves often appear as small triangles (as illus-trated), but fine, additional lines may sometimes be seen extending from the non-ureter corners of the triangle; retrograde filling of normal renal pelvic diverticula may also be observed. The author used to use compression of the caudal abdomen in the belief that this improved the radiographic evaluation of the renal pelves, but he no longer considers this to be necessary. With experience in interpretation, abdominal compression is not required. The normal ureters usually appear as broken lines. This is perfectly normal and is due to ureteral peristaltic waves, which originate in the renal pelves. The five minute radio-graph is useful for detecting renal pelvic abdormalities (dilation, abnormal masses such as calculi or tumours, pyelitis/pyelonephritis) and lesions of the ureters such as obstruction by calculi and tumours, hydroureter and rupture. It is of little value in the diagnosis of ureteral ectopia (apart from demonstrating any associated hydroureter/hydronephrosis or pyelonephritis).

(**43**) The animal is placed in right lateral recumbency and a lateral radiograph made, centred on the umbilicus, ten minutes after administration of contrast medium. As well as providing an alternative view of the kidneys, the distal ureters can now be seen. If one is fortunate, the ureters will be seen emptying into the urinary bladder, as illustrated. While this is facilitated by the degree of contrast between the positive contrast-filled distal ureters and the air-filled bladder, and also by the fact that the colon and rectum are now empty of faeces, a certain amount of luck is involved. Unless one happens to make an exposure just as a ureteral peristaltic wave propels urine through the distal ureter into the bladder, the termination of the ureter may not be seen. The availability of radio-graphic screening facilities overcomes this problem; however, if this is not available, several consecutive radiographs may have to be made before the termi-nations of the ureters can be seen. In addition, if the bladder neck is intrapelvic, as in this bitch, it may be difficult to decide if the ureters are terminating beyond the bladder neck, hence the necessity for the next film.

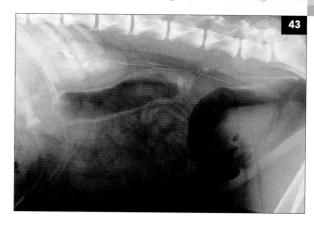

(**44**) Fifteen minutes after administration of contrast medium, a right lateral radiograph is made, centred just cranial to the greater trochanter of the hip and ensuring that the perineum is included on the radiograph.

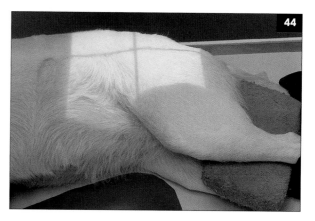

(**45**) The 15 minute film is made mainly to examine for the location of the bladder neck and the presence of ureteral ectopia. Leakage of urine from the bladder may be observed and this may suggest other abnor-malities that require further investigations using retrograde techniques. For example, urine leaking into the urethra may demonstrate the presence of abnormal diverticula or outline radiolucent masses.

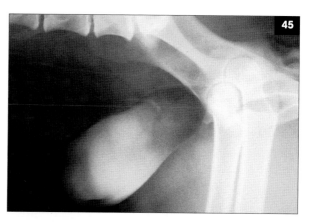

46 The radiographs obtained in **36–45** are usually sufficient in most animals, but in some cases further radiographs will be required, some at different times and/or in different positions (e.g. oblique views). In this example, a radiograph has been made 24 hours after administration of contrast medium to show the grossly dilated ureter and kidney of the dog with hydroureter and hydronephrosis illustrated previously (**19, 32, 33**). In such cases, poor renal excretion into a large volume of residual urine make the normal IVU timings inappropriate.

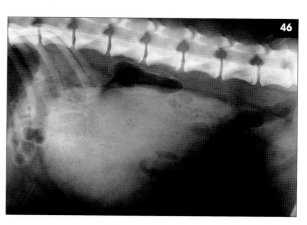

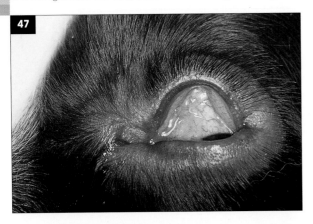

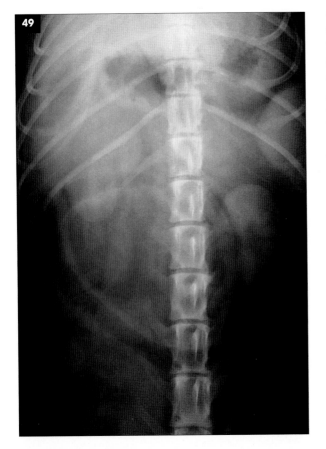

Problems

ADVERSE REACTIONS to the contrast medium occur uncommonly. In lightly anaesthetized or conscious animals, vomiting may occur immediately after administration of contrast medium. Although this is transient, it underlines the need for adequate starvation of the animal prior to general anaesthesia, the use of an endotracheal tube during maintenance of anaesthesia, and an adequate depth of anaesthesia (unless the patient is debilitated or sick).

Other adverse reactions to the contrast medium are anaphylaxis (**47, 48**) and acute renal shutdown (**49**).

47, 48 Anaphylactic reactions to contrast media can occur and were manifested in this Springer Spaniel as acute palpebral oedema (**47**) and in this Boxer as acute urticaria (**48**). Such reactions are obviously more serious if they are more generalized, especially if lung oedema develops. Fortunately, they are extremely rare (these are the only two examples the author has experienced in 37 years) and if they do occur, they respond rapidly to intravenous hydrocortisone.

49 Acute renal shutdown is an unusual complication of IVU. Following administration of contrast medium, a nephrogram is obtained but the ureters fail to be opacified. The nephrogram persists, with no evidence of further excretion, as shown in this radiograph made 15 minutes after administration of contrast medium. This problem can be successfully treated by diuresing the animal using intravenous fluids (normal saline or glucose-saline) combined with intravenous frusemide.

Retrograde, positive contrast vagino-urethrography

Indications

- Vaginal abnormalities, particularly where these prevent physical examinations.
- Suspected urethral lesions.
- Dysuric female dogs and cats.
- Incontinent female dogs and cats.
- Assessment of urethral length and bladder neck position in bitches with suspected urethral sphincter mechanism incompetence.

Some indications for the use of this technique are illustrated (**50–53**). In incontinent bitches with a suspected diagnosis of urethral sphincter mechanism incompetence, vagino-urethrography is the preferred radiographic method of assessing urethral length and bladder neck position, since it is the technique least likely to alter these parameters.

50, 51 Extensive vaginal neoplasia in this bitch (**50**) prevented adequate digital or endoscopic examinations. Vagino-urethrography (**51**) was used to determine the sites and extent of the tumours before surgical intervention.

52 Vagino-urethrography demonstrates marked urethral irregularity in this dog with urethral malignancy. If urethrography had been performed, part of the lesion would have been obscured by the catheter used to introduce contrast medium.

53 In this example, vagino-urethrography has been used to demonstrate the termination of an ectopic ureter in the distal urethra. This might have been missed during urethrography if the urethral catheter cuff was obscuring the ureteral orifice. In addition, urethrography alone fails to demonstrate vaginal terminations of ectopic ureters.

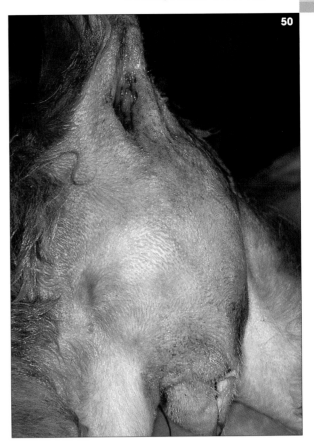

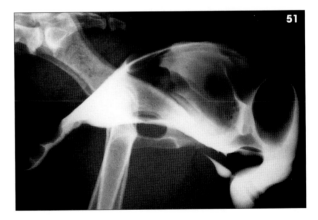

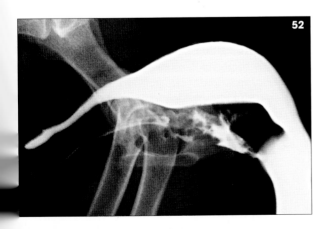

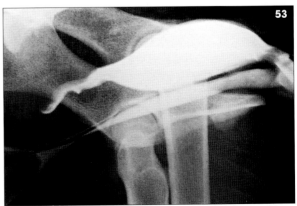

Technique

THE PATIENT SHOULD BE prepared as for an IVU (see p.20). General anaesthesia is required for vagino-urethrography. The radiographic positioning is shown in **44** and, as with any contrast radiographic technique, a plain film of the area should be made first. Air can be used as a contrast medium, but water-soluble iodine-based positive contrast media are preferable. The technique is illustrated below (**54–59**).

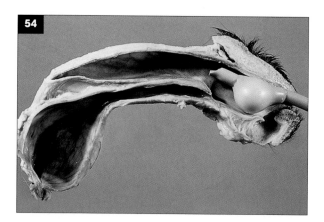

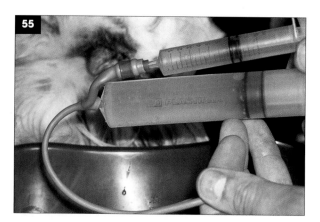

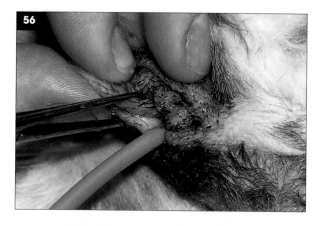

54 The principle of vagino-urethrography is that contrast medium is introduced into the vestibule, usually using a Foley catheter. Once the vagina is filled, contrast enters the urethra. The advantage of this technique over urethrography is that the whole length of the urethra is demonstrated without the presence of a catheter, which might obscure or distort a lesion.

55 As with any retrograde radiographic contrast technique, the catheter should be filled with contrast medium before being inserted. If this is not done, air bubbles may be introduced into the urethra and can be misdiagnosed as calculi or tumours. The Foley catheter is designed to take a wide-nozzle syringe or adapter, but this end of the catheter can be trimmed to allow a Luer syringe nozzle to be attached directly. Approximately 1 ml/kg body weight is required to fill the vagina to the point when the urethra begins to fill. This volume is larger in entire bitches than in spayed bitches and is less if the bitch is incontinent. It is also larger if the bitch is under the influence of endo-genous or exogenous sex hormones, particularly oestrogens, and in incontinent bitches any oestrogen therapy should be discontinued for at least one month before vagino-urethrography (see **60**). Unlike the situation in IVU, the contrast medium is seen undiluted on the radiograph and so a high iodine content is unnecessary. Solutions containing approxi-mately 150 mg iodine equivalent per ml are suitable. The syringe is filled with a volume of contrast medium equivalent to 2 ml/kg body weight. The second syringe is used to inflate the Foley catheter cuff. An 8Fr catheter is suitable for cats and toy breeds of dog and a 10Fr catheter for most other sizes of patient. In animals with short and/or narrow vaginas, especially cats, it is useful to remove the tip of the Foley catheter to facilitate adequate insertion.

56 The Foley catheter cuffed tip is inserted into the vestibule and the cuff inflated. Very little air is required in the cuff of Foley catheters used in cats (0.5–1.0 ml), but the volume of air needed to inflate the cuff in dogs varies from 5 ml (5–15 kg dog) to 10 ml (15–40 kg dog). The cuff should be inflated sufficiently to prevent contrast medium escaping from the vagina, around the catheter. However, over-inflation should be avoided to prevent the inflated cuff from obstructing the external urethral orifice, thus impeding flow of contrast medium. The vulva is then closed caudal to the inflated cuff to prevent the catheter leaving the vagina during filling (the inflated cuff alone is often insufficient to prevent this). The author uses two Allis tissue forceps in bitches and one in cats for this purpose. The first tissue forcep is laced just ventral to the catheter, which is against the orsal commisure of the vulval lips. It is important nat the animal is adequately anaesthetized for agino-urethrography in order to prevent artefacts see **62**). Toleration of Allis tissue forcep placement vithout response is one sign that it is!

7 Once the second tissue forcep has been applied, ontrast medium can be introduced into the vagina. he radiographic exposure is made during the njection of the last quarter of the calculated dose. f fluoroscopic screening facilities are available, the xposure is made once the urethra is adequately filled. f such facilities are not available, it is safest to inject ml/kg body weight and make an exposure during ne last part of the injection. The resultant film can be xamined and, if urethral filling has not occurred, may ive an impression of how much more contrast nedium is required. It is best to fill incrementally, xposing the film during each injection until adequate rethral filling is obtained. This is to avoid the possi-ility of damage to the lower urogenital tract due to verdistension or introduction of large volumes of ontrast medium into ectopic ureters (in incontinent nimals), with possible resultant renal pelvic damage.

58 A vagino-urethrogram in a normal Standard Poodle. There is often a narrowing at the junction between vestibule and vagina, just cranial to the xternal urethral orifice, but in approximately a quarter of bitches, a stricture or perforate hymen may be detected at this site. The dorsal midline filling defects in the cranial vagina are normal and represent dorsal midline folds in the paracervical region. These are more prominent in entire bitches and in entire or neutered bitches under the influence of sex hormones, particularly oestrogens. They should not be confused with vaginal tumours. The urethra usually appears to be widest in its caudal quarter and, sometimes, urethral folds are delineated by the contrast medium as longitudinal striations. The apparent filling defect in he bladder is an artefact due to indentation by adjacent viscera. If the bladder was adequately filled, his artefact would disappear.

59 A normal feline vagino-urethrogram. Note the narrow, short vagina and the long urethra (compared vith the bitch).

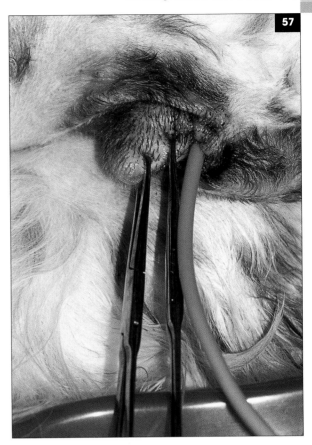

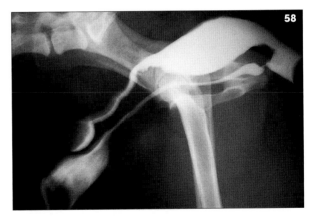

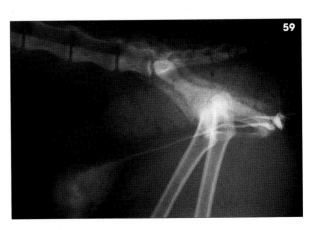

Problems

THERE ARE FEW problems associated with vagino-urethrography (60–62) and most can be avoided using a correct technique (see 54–59). There is a theoretical risk of introducing vaginal and/or urethral organisms into the bladder. However, the author has used this technique on over 1,000 bitches, without the use of prophylactic antibiotics, and has not encountered the problem of urinary tract infection after vagino-urethrography.

60 Vagino-urethrography should not be performed in bitches under the influence of endogenous or exogenous sex hormones. This is particularly true of incontinent bitches that are being treated with oestrogens. The vagina of such animals requires considerably more contrast medium to fill it. The result is that by the time the vagina is full enough for urethral filling to commence, the urethra is under pressure from the distended vagina, contrast medium cannot pass cranially down the urethra and urethral lesions may remain undetected. In addition, the abnormally distended intrapelvic vagina displaces the bladder cranially, making interpretation of bladder neck position inaccurate in bitches with suspected urethral sphincter mechanism incompetence. A distended rectum can have the same effect, underlining the need for the use of an enema before contrast radiography.

61 If vagino-urethrography is performed at the end of an IVU study, care should be taken not to misinterpret ureteral filling due to the IVU as that resulting from reflux of contrast medium introduced during vagino-urethrography. In this example, the distal ureter is overlying the contrast-filled cranial vagina. This may be misdiagnosed as a ureterovaginal fistula. However, apart from the fact that if such a fistula was present the distal ureter would be dilated, retrograde filling would result in denser filling of the ureter compared with the filling due to the more diluted contrast medium of the IVU. In addition, care should be taken not to overfill the Foley catheter cuff or to insert the catheter too far into the vagina, as is the case in this bitch. The result is that the contrast medium is unable to overflow from the vagina into the urethra; therefore, if sufficient contrast medium is introduced, iatrogenic vaginal rupture can occur.

62 It is important that the animal is adequately anaesthetized for vagino-urethrography. If this is not the case, contraction of the constrictor vestibuli muscles may occur, giving the appearance of a vestibulovaginal stricture, as illustrated. The urethralis muscle also contracts, preventing urethral filling. Under adequate anaesthesia, the bitch will not respond to the placement of tissue forceps on the vulva (see 56, 57).

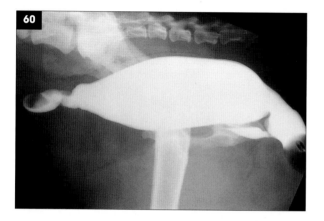

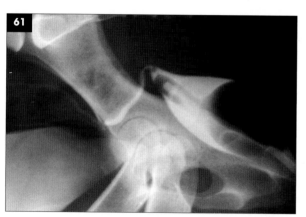

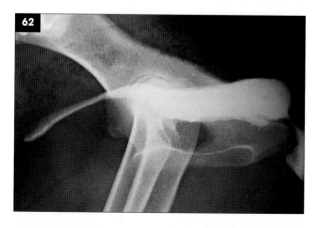

Retrograde, positive contrast urethrography

Indications

- Suspected urethral lesions in male dogs and cats.
- Suspected urethral lesions in female animals in which vagino-urethrography fails adequately to demonstrate the urethra.
- Dysuric animals.
- Incontinent animals.
- Animals with urethral discharges.
- Animals with suspected prostatic disease.

Some indications for the use of retrograde, positive contrast urethrography are illustrated (**63–69**).

63 Urethral lesions are well defined by positive contrast retrograde urethrography. In this cat the technique demonstrates accurately the site and extent of urethral rupture, essential information in deciding the best form of treatment.

64, 65 The additional time spent on contrast radiography is seldom wasted. In this dysuric Pug a plain radiograph had demonstrated the ischial urethral calculus (**64**). This prevented the passage of a urethral catheter, but a retrograde, double contrast urethrocystogram (**65**) revealed that the prognosis was much worse than that associated with urolithiasis. In addition to the urethral calculus, this dog has a transitional cell carcinoma of the bladder neck extending into the pelvic urethra.

66 Urethrography performed in a dysuric bitch in which vagino-urethrography failed to outline the urethra (some contrast medium from the attempted vagino-urethrogram remains in the vagina). A destructive urethral carcinoma is present and was compressed by the vagina as contrast medium was introduced for vagino-urethrography, thus preventing urethral filling. The urethrogram demonstrates the destructive nature of the disease, although the caudal urethra is obscured by the catheter used to introduce the contrast medium. In the presence of a less extensive lesion, a biopsy may be required to differentiate neoplasia from urethritis, since both can have similar contrast radiographic appearances (see **52** and **140**).

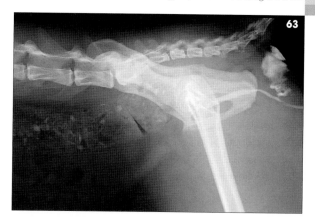

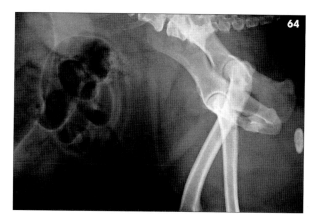

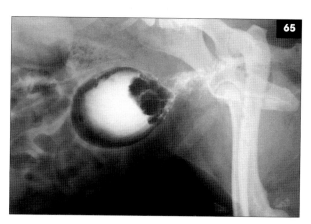

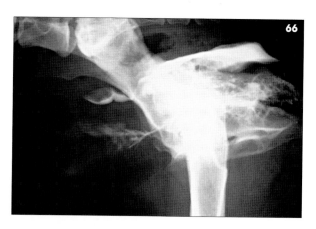

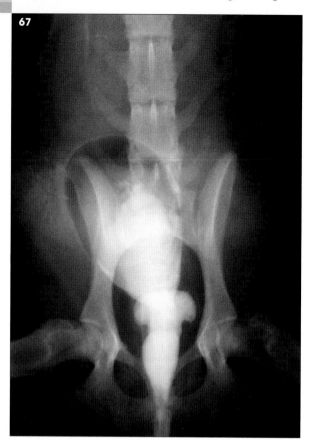

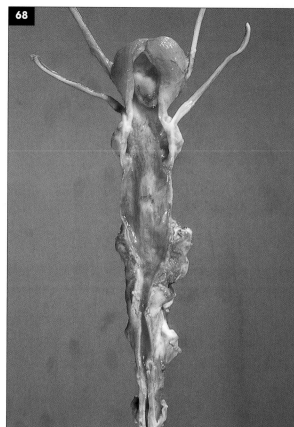

67, 68 (**67**) Urethrography is useful in incontinent male animals. In this example, congenital prostatic urethral diverticulae are demonstrated in an incontinent juvenile male Golden Retriever. The postmortem appearance is shown (**68**).

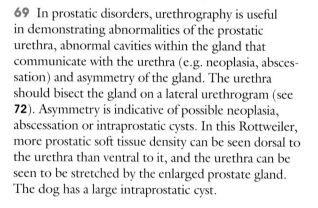

69 In prostatic disorders, urethrography is useful in demonstrating abnormalities of the prostatic urethra, abnormal cavities within the gland that communicate with the urethra (e.g. neoplasia, abscessation) and asymmetry of the gland. The urethra should bisect the gland on a lateral urethrogram (see **72**). Asymmetry is indicative of possible neoplasia, abscessation or intraprostatic cysts. In this Rottweiler, more prostatic soft tissue density can be seen dorsal to the urethra than ventral to it, and the urethra can be seen to be stretched by the enlarged prostate gland. The dog has a large intraprostatic cyst.

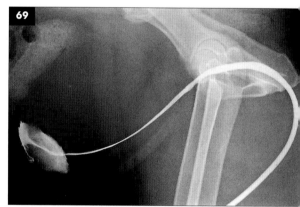

Technique

THE PATIENT should be prepared as for an IVU (see p. 2). General anaesthesia is required for retrograde urethrography. The radiographic positioning is as illustrated in **44**, but in male dogs an additional radiograph should be made centred over the penile/ischial urethra with the hindlimbs flexed cranially (see **26**). As with any contrast radiographic technique, plain films of the area should be made first. Air can be used as a contrast medium, but water-soluble, iodine-based positive contrast media are preferable.

The technique varies slightly between dogs (**70–72**) and cats (**73, 74**) because of the small size of the feline urethra, which does not allow the use of a Foley catheter.

If sufficient contrast medium is introduced, a urethrocystogram can be obtained (see also Cystography, p. 32).

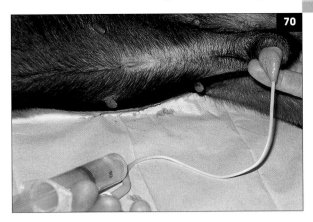

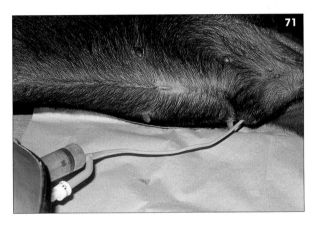

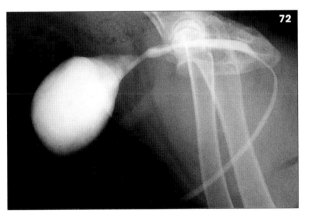

70–72 (**70**) In male dogs, the tip of an 8Fr Foley catheter, which has been pre-filled with contrast medium, is inserted into the penile urethra. As in vagino-urethrography, the Foley catheter can be trimmed to allow direct insertion of the nozzle of a Luer fitting syringe. The volume of contrast medium that will be required varies from approximately 5 ml in toy dogs to 30 ml in giant breeds. The cuff of the catheter is inflated with air to prevent leakage of contrast medium from the distal urethra; approximately 1–5 ml of air is sufficient for dogs from 5–30 kg body weight.

(**71**) The dog is then positioned for radiography. For the pelvic and ischial urethra, the position shown in **44** is suitable, but for suspected lesions of the penile urethra, the hindlimbs should be flexed cranially, as illustrated in **26**, and the X-ray beam centred on the area of interest. As in vagino-urethrography, the radiograph should be made while the urethra is distended with contrast medium. This is accomplished by making the radiographic exposure as the last quarter of the estimated amount of medium is being introduced.

(**72**) In a normal dog the penile urethra is fairly uniform in outline and diameter, but the urethra usually narrows as it passes round the ischial arch. The pelvic urethra is usually wider than the distal urethra, but the appearance of the urethra as it passes through the prostate is variable. Although its outline should be smooth, there is often some variation in the diameter and, sometimes, urethral folds can be seen as longitudinal striations in the contrast column. In a normal dog the urethra should perfectly bisect the prostate on the lateral radiograph.

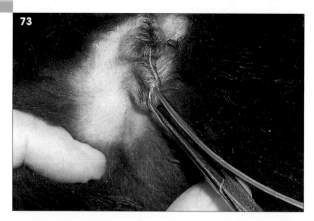

73

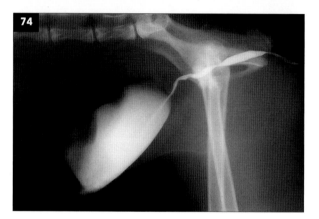

74

Cystography

Indications
- Location of bladder when not visible on plain radiographs.
- Suspected bladder lesions.
- Incontinent animals.
- Dysuric animals.
- Animals with haematuria.

Some examples of indications for cystography are illustrated (**75–79**).

75, 76 Retrograde positive contrast urethro-cystography (**75**) in an Old English Sheepdog with a bilateral perineal rupture and an inguinal hernia (**76**). The urethrocystogram shows that the bladder, which was not visible on plain abdominal films, is in the inguinal hernia rather than the perineal rupture. In such cases, urethrocystography is preferable to cystography since, if the bladder is displaced, the urethra may be kinked and attempts to catheterize the bladder may result in iatrogenic urethral damage (see also Chapter 4, Non-prostatic dysuria).

73 Urethrography in male cats is identical to that in dogs, except that the small diameter of the urethra precludes the use of a Foley catheter. A 3Fr or 4Fr cat catheter is therefore inserted into the penile urethra. To prevent leakage but avoid the risk of penile trauma, the prepuce (not the penis) is occluded around the catheter using Allis tissue forceps.

74 The urethrogram of a normal male cat. The penile urethra is much narrower than the membranous (pelvic) urethra and the urethra narrows again as it passes through the prostate.

Problems
THE PROBLEM OF air in the catheter being introduced with the contrast medium and air bubbles being misdiagnosed as tumours or urethral calculi has been mentioned under the description of vagino-urethrography.

Iatrogenic damage to the lower urinary tract is rare unless complete urethral obstruction is present or an excessive amount of contrast medium is used (see **81**). As with any retrograde technique, there is the potential for introducing organisms, in this case into the proximal urethra or bladder. In practice, and with good technique, the risk of this happening appears to be slight.

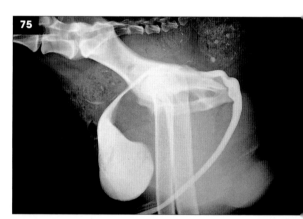

75

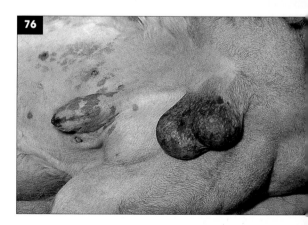

76

77 The site of bladder rupture demonstrated in a male Flat-coated Retriever by retrograde positive contrast urethrocystography. Urethrocystography is preferable to cystography alone in traumatized cases because of the possibility that the urethra may be damaged. Passage of a catheter into the bladder and cystography alone would not demonstrate such damage.

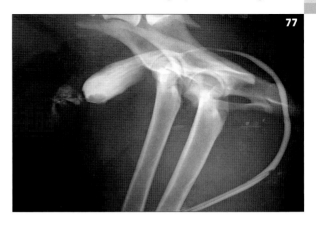

78, 79 (**78**) Transitional cell carcinoma of the bladder neck demonstrated by double contrast cystography in a Corgi. An IVU had also been performed to determine if there was any ureteral involvement in the neoplasia. The tumour has retained positive contrast medium and is clearly outlined by the surrounding air. Although the tumour is close to the trigone, there is no evidence that the ureters or adjacent bladder wall are involved in the neoplasia, an important pre-operative consideration.
(**79**) This dog was euthanased and the postmortem appearance of the tumour can be seen. (NB: This dog has an enlarged prostate due to castration and excessive treatment with oestrogens, leading to squamous metaplasia of the gland).

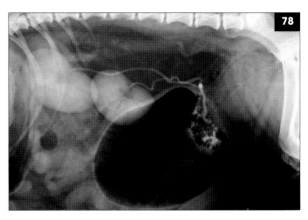

Technique

NEGATIVE, POSITIVE and double contrast techniques are applicable to the urinary bladder. Plain radiographs should be made first. It may be necessary to compare these with the cystogram(s) but, also, the contrast medium may obscure abnormalities such as calculi, which are usually best seen on plain radiographs.

Negative contrast medium is usually air, although other gases such as carbon dioxide can be used. In the author's experience, negative contrast cystography is of little value apart from improving radiographic contrast during IVU and demonstrating gross bladder lesions or bladder position. It is unsuitable for assessing the position of the bladder in bitches with suspected urethral sphincter mechanism incompetence, as the air-filled urinary bladder tends to 'float' and, on lateral projections, often appears to be located further cranially than it actually is. This can be misleading if one is trying to determine if the bladder neck is intrapelvic or not. Negative contrast cystography is a poor technique for demonstrating subtle bladder urothelial abnormalities.

Positive contrast cystography (using the same contrast media as used in vagino-urethrography and urethrography) is useful for demonstrating bladder ruptures (**77**) and diverticula, but it may obscure other abnormalities such as urothelial tumours or vesical calculi.

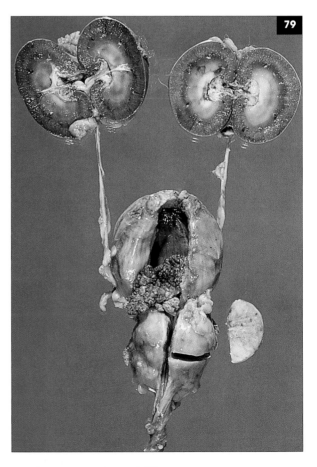

The best technique is to perform retrograde positive contrast urethrography (or vagino-urethrography in female animals) and then to catheterize and empty the bladder of most of the positive contrast medium that has been introduced. The bladder is then filled with air via the same catheter to obtain a double contrast cystogram (**80**). This has the advantage that no lesions are obscured by positive contrast medium, but this contrast medium adheres to bladder urothelial abnormalities and radiolucent calculi, which then are seen clearly against the surrounding negative contrast medium.

80 A normal double contrast cystogram. Most of the positive contrast medium that entered the bladder during urethrography has been removed (it is almost impossible to remove all of it). The bladder has then been filled with air. The volume required varies considerably and it is difficult and inadvisable to give 'dose rates'. Bladder volume varies between animals of different and even the same sizes and the volume required adequately to fill the bladder, while not leading to iatrogenic bladder rupture and/or vesico-ureteral reflux, has yet to be determined. The bladder should be palpated during filling and filled until it begins to feel turgid. It is best to err on the side of caution, make a radiograph and introduce more contrast medium if required. Contrast medium can be introduced via polyurethane catheters or using the softer Foley catheters (see Chapter 3, Urethral catheterization). However, the cuff of the Foley catheter should not be inflated. The inflated cuff may obscure bladder neck lesions and make interpretation difficult. In addition, it may obstruct the ureteral orifices if overinflated and will also prevent air leaking from the bladder around the catheter. In some instances (e.g. a bitch with poor urethral sphincter tone) this may be useful in allowing adequate inflation of the bladder, but it also increases the risk of iatrogenic bladder rupture. If an IVU is being performed at the same time, the positive contrast medium entering the bladder from the ureters can track along the outside of the inflated Foley catheter cuff and resemble an ectopic ureter on subsequent radiographs.

Problems

RARELY, PNEUMOCYSTOGRAPHY has been associated with fatal air embolism. This is more likely if bladder wall damage is present. Other problems are iatrogenic bladder rupture or/and vesico-ureteral reflux (**81**) and misdiagnoses of vesical masses (**82**), or bladder wall thickening (**83, 84**) when neither are present. The latter is most likely if the bladder is inadequately filled with contrast medium.

81 Iatrogenic bladder rupture and vesico-ureteral reflux in a West Highland White Terrier puppy during retrograde positive contrast urethrocystography. Unknown to the author, this dog had bladder hypoplasia, and a relatively small amount of contrast medium was required to cause the damage illustrated. This type of bladder rupture usually takes the form of several urothelial slits through which contrast finds its way into the peritoneal cavity. It is difficult to find the defects in the detrusor muscle through which the contrast has leaked and these do not usually overlie the urothelial slits. Obviously, prevention by careful cystography is best but, if iatrogenic rupture occurs, it can be treated by using an indwelling vesical catheter for 7–10 days until the bladder has healed.

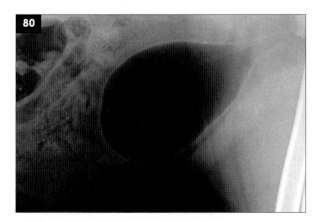

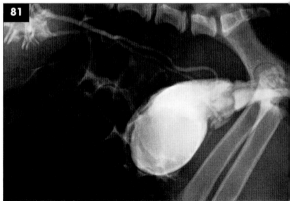

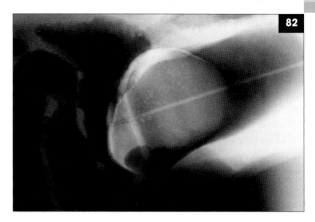

82 'Cerate' calculi demonstrated by double contrast cystography in a dog. 'Cerate' calculi are the result of the previous insertion of a cattle intramammary preparation into the bladder. The same artefacts can be generated by using oil-based lubricants on the urinary catheter used to introduce the contrast medium.

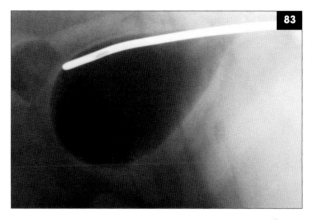

83, 84 Apparent thickening of the bladder wall due to inadequate bladder filling (**83**). One hundred ml of air has been instilled into the bladder, the wall of which appears thickened, especially ventrally. When a further 100 ml of air is introduced, the apparent bladder wall thickening disappears (**84**). The use of a metal catheter, as in this case, is not recommended; apart from the increased risk of iatrogenic catheter damage, the radiodense catheter may obscure a significant lesion. Other artefacts can be due to adjacent viscera, such as loops of small intestine, which may indent the wall of an inadequately filled bladder. Such apparent thickening and/or indentations disappear as further air is introduced (compare **83** with **84**), illustrating the need for adequate bladder filling during cystography.

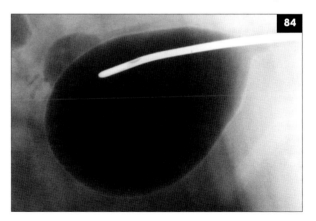

3 Other diagnostic aids

With a little help from my friends
John Lennon (1940–1980) and Paul McCartney (1942–)

IN THIS CHAPTER, other aids to diagnosis in small animals with suspected urological abnormalities are presented. These include ultrasonography, urethral catheterization, fluid collection and examination, biopsy techniques, blood and urine analyses and urodynamics. More specialized procedures such as scintigraphy and MRI or CT scanning are not described here.

Ultrasonography

ULTRASONOGRAPHY has revolutionized the diagnosis of urological disorders. It is the perfect partner to good radiography, since the contrast of ultrasound pictures is often best at times when radiographic contrast is reduced, for example in the presence of fluid. It is particularly useful in demonstrating abnormalities of the internal architecture of soft tissue organs and in the diagnosis and localization of collections of fluid within or around viscera. It is especially helpful in the differentiation of prostatic disorders, especially cysts and abscesses. Ultrasonography allows accurate localization of a lesion so that meaningful and safer (ultrasound-guided) biopsy or fluid samples can be obtained.

Indications
ANY SUSPECTED ABNORMALITIES of urinary tract viscera suggested by clinical or/and radiographic investigations (**85–86** and **255–263**).

85 Hydronephrosis demonstrated ultrasonographically in a dog. The black, anechoic centre represents the fluid (f) in the dilated renal pelvis. This is surrounded by the hypoechoic, dark grey renal parenchyma within which can be seen an area of hyperechoic, white tissue (arrowed). This may represent the fibrous tissue of the wall of the renal pelvis or scarring within the kidney parenchyma.

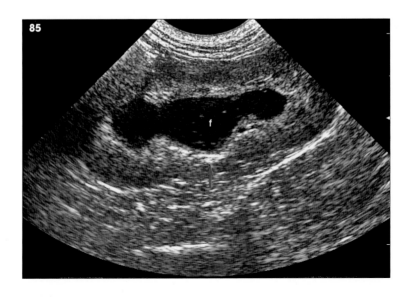

86 Ultrasound-guided centesis of the prostate. Ultrasonography allows needles to be inserted accurately into quite small intraprostatic cysts and abscesses for drainage of fluid for cytology, bacteriology, etc. It can also be used to guide biopsy needles into urinary tract organs and to ensure that the region to be biopsied is not fluid-filled (e.g. an abscess), thus reducing the risk of peritonitis.

Technique

ULTRASONOGRAPHIC PRACTICE and interpretation requires considerable expertise, based on experience. The would-be veterinary ultrasonographer is referred to the latest reworking of Frances Barr's excellent book on the subject by Paddy Mannion (2006) and the descriptions that follow are merely overviews of the use of ultrasonography in the urinary tract (**87–88**).

In the urinary tract, real-time B mode ultrasonography is most commonly employed to examine the internal structure of the kidneys, bladder and prostate. The patient preparation is the same for all organs and involves clipping of the coat from the area to be scanned, cleaning the skin with surgical spirit to remove dirt and grease, and application of liberal quantities of commercial accoustic gel to ensure good contact between the skin and transducer.

The urinary bladder and prostate are imaged from a prepubic (in the case of male dogs, parapenile) site, as used in the dog shown in **86**. Rectal ultrasonography of the prostate is possible in large dogs, but requires a transducer specifically designed for rectal work.

87, 88 The kidneys are usually imaged from the flanks. (**87**) The site for the left kidney is just caudal to the last rib, ventral to the sublumbar muscles (cranial is to the left in this illustration). (**88**) The right kidney is further cranial and so is imaged between the last two or three ribs on the right (cranial is to the right in this illustration). However, the presence of the ribs means that accoustic shadows due to the ribs may be cast on the renal image, preventing the whole kidney from being imaged at once.

Problems

THERE ARE FEW problems associated with ultrasonography of the urinary tract apart from those encountered in technique and interpretation due to inexperience. The presence of the ribs can lead to difficulties imaging the right kidney and similar problems are encountered if gas-filled bowel is interspaced between the transducer and the organ being imaged.

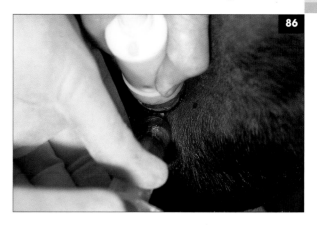
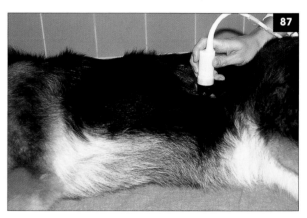
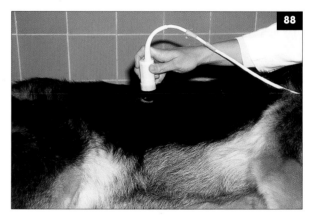

Urethral catheterization

Indications
- To obtain urine samples for laboratory analyses.
- To relieve dysuria (**89**).
- To provide urinary by-pass (e.g. urethral injuries) or drainage (e.g. bladder paralysis) (**90–91**).
- To detect urethral obstruction (inaccurate – see **139**).
- To introduce contrast media into the urinary tract.

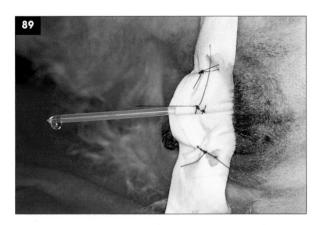

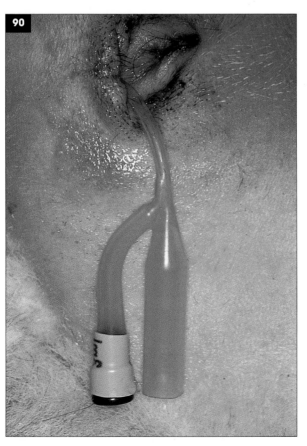

89 A catheter can be used temporarily to relieve dysuria, allowing the animal to recover from the systemic consequences and the local effects on the bladder of urinary obstruction before the cause is treated. While passage of a urethral catheter is suitable in cases of neurogenic dysuria or obstruction by soft tissue masses, it should be performed with care in cases of suspected urolithiasis. Attempts forcibly to pass a catheter in such cases are likely to result in iatrogenic urethral trauma (see **107–110**). Foley catheters can be used in animals without urethral obstruction (see **90**), but they may be difficult to pass in animals with urethral narrowing, are too large for cats and are sometimes not long enough for large male dogs. Polyurethane catheters can be used for the short-term relief of dysuria. Once the bladder has been drained, the catheter can be sutured *in situ* and maintained as an indwelling catheter until the animal is fit for elective surgery, if this is necessary to treat the cause of the dysuria. In dogs the catheter can be fixed to the perivulval (in bitches, as illustrated) or cranial preputial (in male dogs) skin using a butterfly tape made from adhesive dressing.

90 A Foley catheter can be used as an indwelling catheter, provided that it can be passed along the urethra. If this is not possible, a prepubic tube cystostomy catheter can be used for urinary bypass (see **231–234**). Any urine obtained should be submitted for laboratory examination. Urine samples are useful in the differential diagnosis of the cause of dysuria (e.g. cytology in the case of suspected malignancy) and urinary tract infections are common in animals with urinary retention. However, because of the potential for introduction of urethral organisms into the bladder (and thus the urine sample), low bacterial counts in catheterized urine samples are probably insignificant and should be ignored. Ideally, indwelling catheters should be connected to closed urine collecting systems, and this should be the goal. While this is possible in recumbent (e.g. as in **113–114**) or paraplegic patients using, for example, sterile intravenous drip tubing and bags, it may be impracticable in ambulatory patients and the system may have to be left open. In the author's experience, significant urinary tract infections in animals with such open systems are remarkably uncommon, although he routinely uses prophylactic antibiotics in such cases. There is some argument about the use of prophylactic antibiotics, and some authors are concerned that they may lead to proliferation of resistant organisms. Bacteriological cultures of urine and/or the catheter tip are recommended following catheter removal.

91 In dysuric cats the Jackson's catheter is designed for use as an indwelling catheter. Once the catheter has been passed, it is sutured to the prepuce using the holes in the catheter flange. An Elizabethan collar should be fitted to the cat, since many cats are able to detach the catheter from the flange and remove it. Some Jackson's catheters are only just long enough to reach the bladder lumen of male cats. This means that, if the catheter is attached to a closed collecting system, the tip of the catheter may be withdrawn into the cranial urethra (preventing drainage) if the animal is ambulatory and pulls on the collecting system.

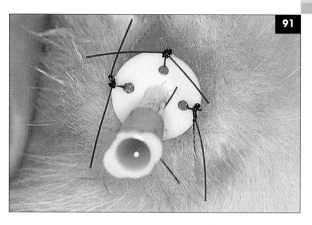

Technique

THE TECHNIQUE VARIES between the sexes and between dogs and cats (**92–105**). Most dogs can be catheterized without chemical restraint, but cats, especially males, usually require sedation or anaesthesia.

92 A variety of catheters are available for urethral catheterization of small animals. In general, polyurethane and Foley catheters are suitable for use in both sexes of dogs and cats, although Foley catheters may be difficult to introduce. The catheter examples illustrated below are, with one exception, suitable for most urological situations in small animals. From left to right they are:

- 12Fr, 10Fr and 8Fr Foley catheters: the 12Fr and 10Fr sizes are suitable for introducing contrast medium during vagino-urethrography and the 10Fr and 8Fr sizes can be used for urethral catheterization and urethrography (the 10Fr in large bitches). Foley catheters may be used as indwelling catheters, although the longer Foley catheters may be difficult to insert in dysuric male dogs, as they tend to bend within the urethra if they meet an obstructive lesion.
- 8Fr and 6Fr polyurethane catheters: suitable for urethral catheterization in large and medium size male and female dogs.
- 3Fr and 4Fr polyurethane catheters: suitable for catheterization of small dogs (the longer catheter) and cats. The right-hand catheter is a Jackson's catheter designed for use as an indwelling catheter in cats.
- A metal bitch catheter: metal catheters are more likely to traumatize the urethra and/or bladder and, in the author's opinion, should never be used.

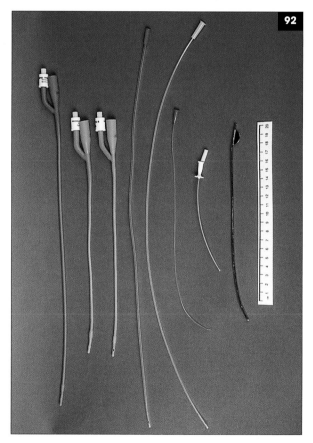

93, 94 In male dogs the caudal os penis is grasped with one hand and the other hand used to retract the prepuce caudally, exposing the glans penis. One of the fingers of the hand holding the penis (the little finger, in this case) is looped dorsal to the retracted prepuce and used to keep the glans exposed whilst the catheter is inserted (**93**). Catheters should be lubricated with sterile, water-soluble jelly and inserted into the urethra under aseptic conditions. The use of oil-based lubricants is inadvisable, particularly if contrast radiography is to be performed (see **82**). The catheter should be handled through its sterile polythene bag (as illustrated) or a sterile surgical glove should be worn on the hand used to insert the catheter. Once the catheter has been inserted to the level of the caudal os penis, the grip of the hand holding the penis is relaxed slightly during further passage of the catheter (this hand may be kinking the urethra, making catheter passage more difficult), as shown (**94**). Passage of the catheter is discontinued as soon as the catheter tip enters the bladder and urine appears at the catheter hub.

95–99 A variety of vaginal specula are available to facilitate passage of a urinary catheter in bitches (e.g. Kilians, Sims and McIntyre specula). The speculum viewed from above in **95** is designed with an open slit which is apposed to the vaginal floor. The speculum is inserted into the vagina, slit side ventrally as shown in **96** (taking care to avoid the clitoral fossa) and the raised external urethral orifice identified on the floor of the vagina, at its junction with the vestibule, as can be seen on this endoscopic view (**97**). The bitch can be positioned in dorsal or lateral recumbency for this procedure. If the dorsal recumbent position is used, the hindlimbs should be flexed and if difficulty is encountered in locating the external urethral orifice with the bitch in this position, catheterization in right lateral recumbency (if one is right-handed; left lateral recumbency if one is left-handed) should be attempted since this is often easier. Location of the external urethral orifice and passage of the catheter is often facilitated if an assistant pulls the ventral vulva caudally (**96**). This has the effect of flattening the vestibular floor, which is advantageous, particularly if there are vestibular and vaginal mucosal folds (these are more pronounced in some breeds [e.g. Bulldogs] or in bitches under the influence of endogenous or exogenous sex hormones). The catheter is then inserted into the urethra aseptically (**98**) and advanced until urine just begins to flow. The view through the speculum of the catheterized external urethral orifice is shown (**99**).

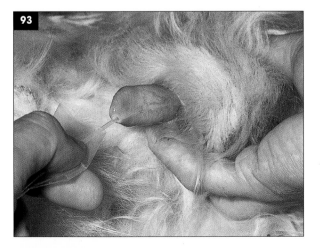

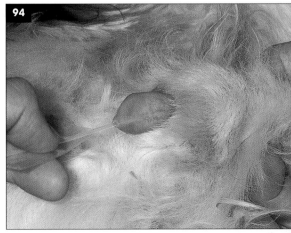

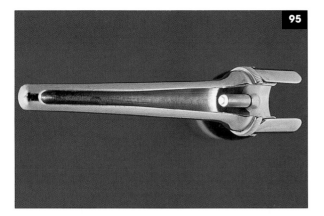

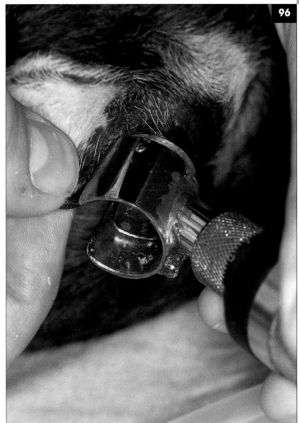

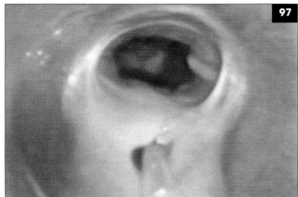

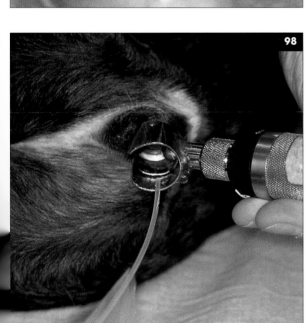

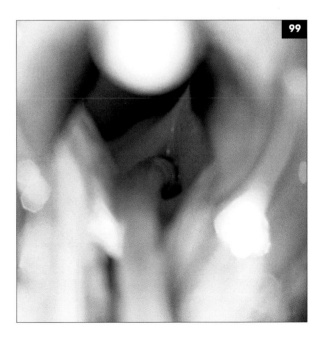

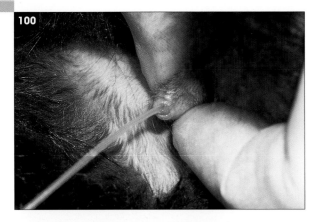

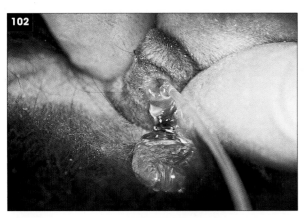

100, 101 (**100**) In male cats the thumb and index finger of the left hand (if one is right-handed) are used to push the prepuce cranially and expose the glans penis. The catheter tip is inserted into the penile urethra. Further attempts at passage at this stage are inadvisable; the left hand fingers almost invariably kink the urethra, making further passage difficult and increasing the risk of iatrogenic urethral trauma.

(**101**) Further passage of the catheter is accomplished by gripping the prepuce with the left hand and pulling it caudally. This has the effect of aligning the penile and membranous urethrae and the catheter can now usually be passed without difficulty.

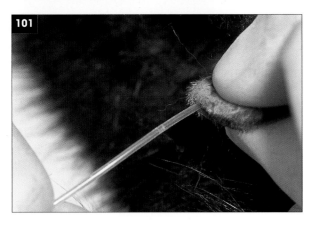

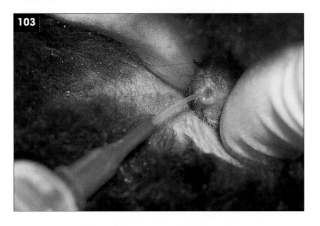

102 In obstructed male cats, urinary catheters are not suitable for flushing calculus material from the penile urethra. It is not usually possible to introduce the catheter so that both side holes are within the penile urethra. Therefore, any flushing liquids merely pass out of the catheter side hole outside the urethra, as illustrated, and fail to dislodge calculus material.

103 Initially, it is better to use a lacrimal cannula to flush the obstructed feline penile urethra. Before doing so, however, it is important that the bladder is emptied of urine by cystocentesis (see p. 45). As well as being part of the pre-operative management of obstructed animals, this will ensure that the flushing fluids are not working against a high intravesical pressure. Once the penile urethra has been cleared, a catheter can then be passed, used to flush remaining calculus from the membranous urethra, and maintained as an indwelling catheter to allow the animal to recover from the effects of the obstruction and to introduce calculus dissolution or flushing fluids into the bladder. In the author's view, it is the flushing itself that dislodges the calculus from the urethra rather than any dissolution by the flushing solution. He therefore prefers to use sterile saline to proprietary solutions such as Walpole's solution, which may irritate an already inflamed urethra.

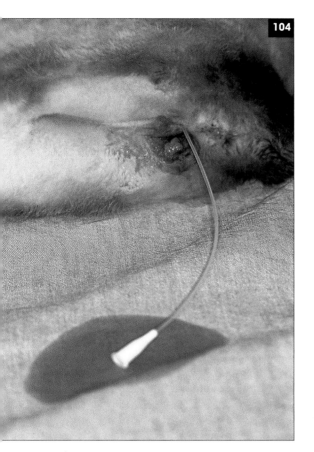

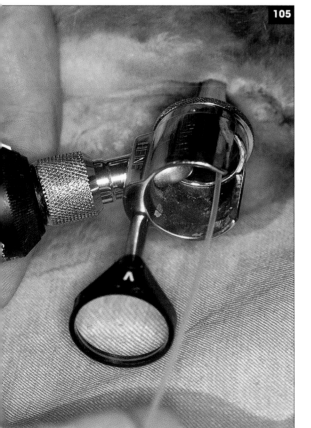

104, 105 Female cats can often be catheterized 'blind'. Unlike the situation in the bitch, the feline external urethral orifice is not raised on a papilla, but is a midline aperture on the vaginal floor. A catheter placed in the midline on the vestibular floor and passed cranially will often enter the urethra (**104**). If this does not happen, an auroscope makes a useful vaginoscope for female cats through which the external urethral orifice can be identified and a catheter passed (**105**).

Problems

URETHRAL CATHETERIZATION is associated with two main problems, both of which can be overcome by attention to technique. These are introduction of organisms into and iatrogenic trauma to the lower urinary tract (**106–110**).

If catheterized urine is to be examined for the presence of blood, the urine should be allowed to flow freely into the sample bottle (**106**).

106 Urine for laboratory analyses (particularly if haematuria is suspected) should be allowed to flow passively from the catheter. Manual compression of the bladder with the catheter *in situ* or suction on the catheter may both result in iatrogenic haematuria, which may lead to misinterpretation of the laboratory results. For this reason, some authors prefer cystocentesis but this can also lead to iatrogenic haematuria.

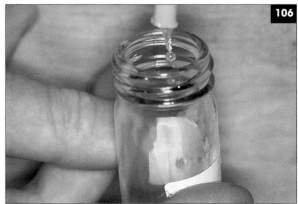

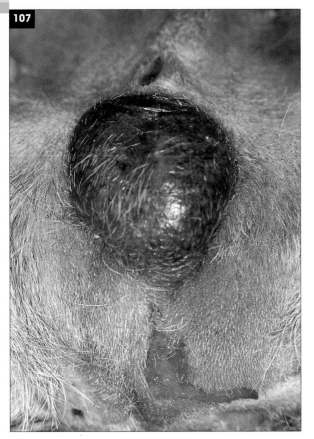

107 Ischial urethral abscess, draining through the perineum, due to attempts to catheterize a dysuric male dog with urolithiasis (this dog had also had a prescrotal urethrotomy). This could have been avoided by attention to aseptic technique and avoidance of excessive pressure during attempts to pass the catheter. If a catheter cannot be passed easily, attempts to pass it should be abandoned and the reason for the apparent urethral obstruction ascertained. A tortuous groove of the os penis may prevent passage of a urinary catheter and feel like an obstruction due to a urethral calculus. In fact, it is of no clinical significance, but this underlines the inadvisability of using a urinary catheter to detect urethral obstruction. If in doubt, urethrography should be performed.

108 If the catheter is introduced too far, it may follow the contour of the bladder wall and begin to exit into the proximal urethra alongside itself. Even worse, it may form a knot inside the bladder. Under these circumstances, the catheter may be very difficult or even impossible to remove via the urethra. The catheter illustrated was passed too far into a dog's bladder via a perineal urethrostomy and became knotted. Fortunately, because of the urethrostomy, it could be removed via the urethra, but this resulted in urethral damage and haemorrhage, as can be seen from the blood clots attached to the catheter.

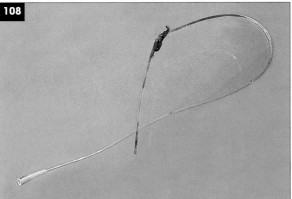

109, 110 Unless severely debilitated, cats should never be catheterized without adequate chemical restraint. The skin loss from the lateral (**109**) and medial (**110**) aspects of this cat's hindlimbs are due to the effect of subcutaneous urine after urethral rupture. The rupture was iatrogenic and due to attempts to catheterize this cat conscious when it became dysuric (because of urethritis) two days after perineal urethrostomy.

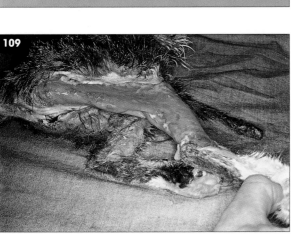

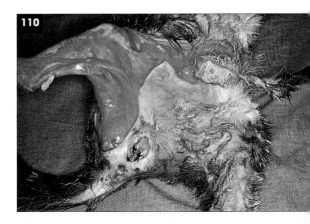

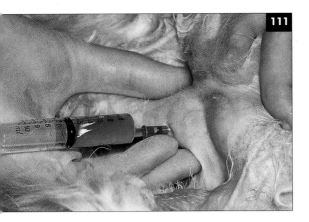

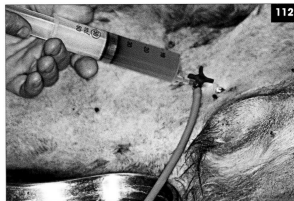

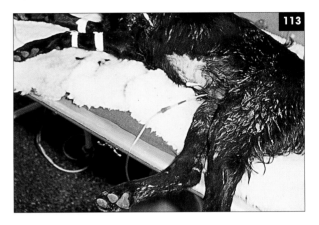

Centesis

Indications

- Collection of fluids for laboratory examinations (**111**).
- Drainage of fluids from the abdomen or urinary tract organs (**112**).

111   Centesis can be used to obtain samples for laboratory examinations. In this example, urine is being obtained from a sick, aged cat for bacteriology. This avoids the need for sedation or anaesthesia for catheterization and, in the view of many veterinary urologists, is the preferred method of obtaining urine samples for bacteriological examinations.

112   In this dysuric dog, cystocentesis is being used as an emergency procedure to drain the urinary bladder (see also **211–213**). In addition to bladder drainage, the metabolic consequences of the dysuria should be corrected; these measures take priority over determination of the cause of the dysuria.

Techniques

THE TECHNIQUE VARIES slightly depending on the site of the fluid; centesis of the abdomen, urinary bladder and prostate gland is described (**113–115**). In all cases, attention should be paid to aseptic and atraumatic technique.

113, 114 (**113**) For abdominocentesis, the author's preferred site is just caudal to the umbilicus: attempts to drain abdominal fluid from sites cranial to the umbilicus usually fail because the end of the draining needle or catheter becomes obstructed by falsiform fat. Fenestrated abdominal drains can be used but, if these are not readily available, large bore (14–18G) over-the-needle cannulae are suitable for abdominocentesis. The bladder can be drained via a prepubic, median (female animals and male cats) or paramedian (male dogs) site and the needle angled caudally towards the bladder neck (see **111**). For bladder emptying, the needle should be inserted into the caudal bladder; otherwise, as the bladder empties it may retract caudally off the needle. A fine (21–25G) needle should be used to reduce the possibility of urine leakage from the puncture site. Cystocentesis is easy to perform if the bladder is palpable, but may be difficult if the bladder is empty and/or caudally positioned, as it may be in cases of bladder rupture and in incontinent bitches. In these cases, ultrasonography is helpful in locating accurately the cystocentesis needle. The Flat-coated Retriever shown in **113** has a ruptured bladder; the urethrocystogram is illustrated in **77**. The dog is not sedated, but rather is collapsed due to the metabolic consequences of uroperitoneum (i.e. hyperkalaemia, acidosis and azotaemia).

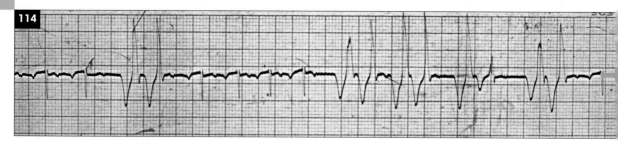

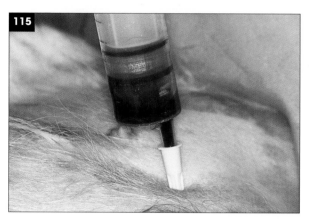

(**114**) The effects of the acidosis and hyperkalaemia on the heart can be appreciated from the ECG. An over-the-needle intravenous cannula has been inserted just caudal to the umbilicus and is being used both to drain urine from and to introduce dialysing fluids into the peritoneal cavity. In this example, abdominocentesis is being used (along with intravenous fluid therapy and the insertion of an indwelling urethral catheter) to relieve the uroperitoneum and its metabolic consequences. Although syringe suction may speed the rate of fluid removal, it is frequently counterproductive, since omentum or other abdominal viscera may be sucked onto the end of the drain/catheter, preventing the exit of fluids. It is often better to allow the fluid to drain passively through the drain/catheter.

115 Large prostatic cysts or abscesses can be drained by centesis (see also **263** and **302**). As well as providing fluid for laboratory examinations, such drainage may also be used as a first aid measure to relieve dysuria and reduce toxaemia (in the case of abscesses), thus allowing the animal to be stabilized before any surgery is performed. The site for centesis is chosen by palpation of the location of the fluid-filled cyst or abscess, although small lesions can be more accurately located using ultrasound (see **86**).

Problems

POTENTIAL PROBLEMS include introduction o infection into the area from which fluid is bein; removed, leakage of fluid from a viscus into the sur rounding tissues or peritoneum, and iatrogenic viscera trauma. The risk of these complications can b minimized by aseptic, atraumatic technique and the us of the smallest needle/cannula compatible with the flui to be removed. For example, urine can be drained from the bladder using fine needles (21–23G), whereas larger bore may be necessary to remove thick, viscou pus from a prostatic abscess or adequately to drain flui from the abdomen. The use of ultrasonography make any attempt at centesis much safer, since the drainin; needle can be placed more accurately (see **263**)

Cytology

Indications

IN UROLOGY, cytology is mainly used to differentiat inflammatory and malignant conditions (**116–117**).

116 Cytology of fluid (H&E x300) obtained by ultrasound-guided centesis from a prostatic cavity of a dog. The large numbers of inflammatory cells and bacteria present suggest a diagnosis of prostatic abscessation or infected prostatic cyst.

117 Cytology of fluid (H&E x300) obtained from a canine prostatic cyst, illustrating the presence of neoplastic cells. This animal had a carcinoma of the cyst lining.

Techniques

CYTOLOGICAL EXAMINATIONS can be performed on cellular material in fluids such as urine, ascitic fluid or prostatic secretions, on that obtained by urethral washings and on material resulting from brushings during endoscopy of the lower urinary tract.

Several smears of the sample should be made on to microscope slides. The retrieval of cells is higher if the smears are made of the material at the bottom of the container after standing or if a cytospin/cytoslide system is used. The slides are then air dried and, in most practice situations, packaged according to mailing regulations and forwarded to a diagnostic laboratory. If such a laboratory is not available and/or a veterinary surgeon with an interest or training in pathology is employed within the practice, the slides may be stained and examined immediately.

A number of staining techniques can be used for cytology, but rapid haematoxylin and eosin and Leishman stains are usually adequate and most likely to be available in general practice. The staining techniques are summarized in *Tables 6* and *7*.

Table 6 **Rapid H & E stain**
1 Fix slide in acetic alcohol (3% acetic acid in 95% alcohol) for one minute.
2 Wash in water.
3 Stain in Harris' haematoxylin for one minute.
4 Wash and 'blue' (wait until the stain turns blue) in running tap water for one minute.
5 Stain in eosin (1% in tap water) for two minutes.
6 Wash in water.
7 Dehydrate in 100% alcohol, rinse in xylene and mount in DPX.
Results: nuclei – blue; other cellular components – shades of red and pink.

Table 7 **Leishman stain**
1 Put slide(s) on a rack and cover with one squirt of Leishman stock (made up of 0.15% Leishman powder in 100% methanol – use within 24 hours); leave for 20 seconds.
2 Add two squirts of pH 6.8 buffer and tip rack up and down to ensure mixing; leave for seven minutes.
3 Rinse quickly in distilled water and recover with pH 6.8 buffer for two minutes.
4 Rinse quickly in distilled water.
5 Blot dry. Do not use alcohol.
6 Clear and mount.

Results:

nuclei	– purple
acidophils	– pink/red
basophils	– blue
eosinophils	– red/orange
mast cells	– purple (granules)

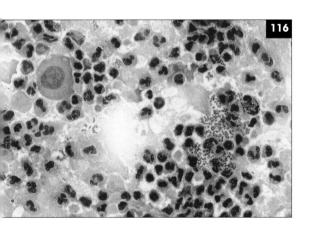

116

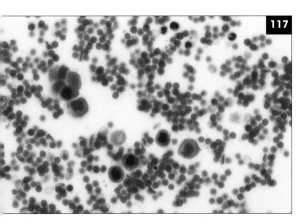

117

Problems

THE PREPARATION of good, diagnostic slides and their interpretation comes only with practice and experience. This is unlikely to be acquired in most practices and so the reader is advised to concentrate on preparing an even, air-dried smear on a slide for staining and interpretation at a veterinary pathological diagnostic laboratory. Even then, the results may be unreliable. In most cases, cytology is being used to differentiate malignant from benign conditions as a guide to treatment and prognosis. While the finding of malignant cells is diagnostic of malignancy, the converse is, unfortunately, not true. The absence of malignant cells on cytology does not exclude a diagnosis of malignancy; such cells are not always found. In the author's experience, cytology is less reliable than the biopsy techniques described below in the differentiation of malignant and non-malignant urological disorders.

Biopsy techniques

Indications

- To differentiate inflammatory and neoplastic lesions of the urinary tract (e.g. urethritis vs urethral carcinoma).
- To determine the nature of the disease present, more accurately to prescribe treatment and/or obtain a prognosis (e.g. malignancies, glomerular renal diseases).

Techniques

ALTHOUGH BIOPSY MATERIAL can be obtained by surgical exposure of the organ concerned, less invasive methods include needle biopsies and biopsies taken endoscopically (see Endoscopy, p. 55) or using a urethral catheter.

The kidney and prostate can be biopsied using a 'Tru-cut' disposable biopsy needle (Travenol) (**118–123**), preferably under ultrasonic guidance, while the catheter biopsy technique (**124–126**) is suitable for lower urinary tract urothelial lesions and the para-urethral prostate.

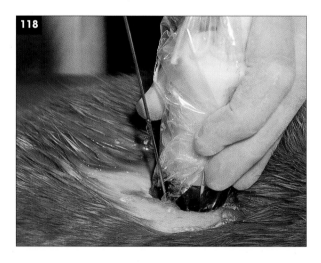

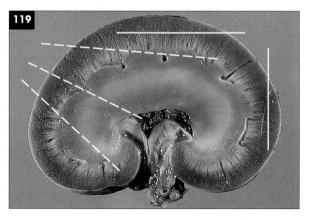

118, 119 (**118**) Renal cortical biopsies can be taken using a biopsy needle. A Tru-cut biopsy needle is being used to take a biopsy of this cat's left kidney. Accurate placement of the needle is necessary in order to obtain a meaningful biopsy while minimizing renal trauma. Therefore, although a biopsy can be taken from a sedated animal using local analgesia, the author prefers to perform the technique under general anaesthesia, if possible. Ideally, biopsy should be performed using an automated Tru-cut biopsy instrument under ultrasound guidance, since this makes the procedure less hazardous for the animal. The skin over the kidney (see **87–88**) is prepared for aseptic surgery and sterile ultrasound gel applied. In this illustration, surgical drapes have been omitted to facilitate orientation. The biopsy needle is inserted through a stab incision in the skin into the renal cortex under ultrasonic guidance and the biopsy taken, in this case using an 18Fr Biopty-cut needle and automatic biopsy 'gun'. If such facilities are not available and a manual Tru-cut needle has to be used, it is important to be familiar with the functioning of the biopsy needle before inserting it. This may seem obvious, but most veterinary surgeons perform needle biopsies infrequently and once the needle has been inserted, the effects of manipulations cannot be seen. The novice is advised to have two needles available; one to take the biopsy and the other in case he/she forgets what to do once the first needle has been inserted! The biopsy needle is introduced via a small stab skin incision and inserted into the kidney cortex, taking care to avoid the medulla or corticomedullary junction. In cats the kidneys are usually sufficiently palpable and mobile to be held through the skin and abdominal wall. The kidneys of dogs, on the other hand, may be difficult to locate and fix adequately and some authors suggest making a small flank incision through which a finger can be inserted into the abdomen, better to fix the kidney. In both species the left kidney is easier to biopsy than the right because of its more caudal location; therefore, this is the author's kidney of choice in cases of generalized renal disease (e.g. glomerulonephropathies). However, other practitioners prefer the right kidney, since this is less mobile than the left. The author prefers to hold the kidney in one hand (the left if one is right-handed) and to insert the needle with the other. Unless one has access to a biopsy 'gun', this means that an assistant is required to manipulate the needle in order to obtain a biopsy. Once the needle is withdrawn, it should be examined to ensure that the amount of tissue obtained is adequate for laboratory examinations (histology, electron microscopy and immunohistochemistry) and pieces of tissue should be transferred to suitable containers.

(**119**) Kidney specimen (from a dog with benign, idiopathic renal haemorrhage) illustrating the correct (solid lines) and incorrect (broken lines) positions of insertion of the biopsy needle.

120–123 (**120**) A needle biopsy of the prostate gland is usually obtained through the perineum, as illustrated in the diagram, but a similar technique can be used prepubically to biopsy an intra-abdominal prostate gland. The prostate is fixed, in the case of trans-perineal biopsy using a gloved finger in the rectum. The finger is also used to guide the needle into the area of the gland to be biopsied. Care is taken to avoid the urethra.

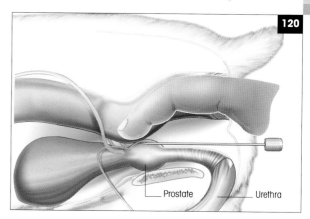

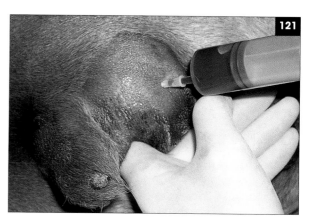

Prostate   Urethra

(**121**) The rectum is evacuated, either by the administration of an enema or by digital removal of faeces. The anaesthetized dog is placed in lateral recumbency with the side to be biopsied uppermost. The perineum is prepared for aseptic surgery and sterile drapes applied, leaving the anus and perineum exposed (the drapes have been removed from this dog to facilitate orientation). The prostate is fixed with the index finger of the left hand (right-handed people). The biopsy needle or needle for centesis (as shown in this Boxer with a prostatic cyst extending caudally into the perineum) is introduced into the perineum adjacent to the anus and above it, as shown. This reduces the risk of contamination of the needle by faecal organisms, since any material leaving the anus will tend to fall downwards, away from the needle. Once the needle is inserted into the prostate, fluids can be withdrawn or a Tru-cut biopsy taken in an identical way to a renal biopsy. The centre of the gland is avoided to prevent iatrogenic prostatic urethral trauma and the biopsy needle is usually inserted into the dorsolateral region of the prostate.

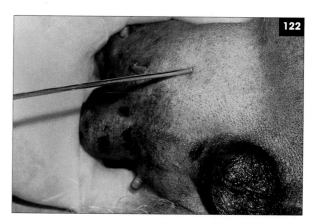

(**122**) If the prostate is cranial to the pubic brim, it can be biopsied via a prepubic approach as shown (again, the surgical drapes have been removed to facilitate orientation). The prostate is fixed with the left hand (if one is right-handed) and the right hand used to introduce the biopsy needle, taking care to avoid the urethra in the centre of the gland.

(**123**) The resulting biopsy is illustrated. The prostatic enlargement, alopecia and feminization in the dog in **122** are due to excessive, prolonged oestrogen therapy, leading to squamous metaplasia of the prostate gland.

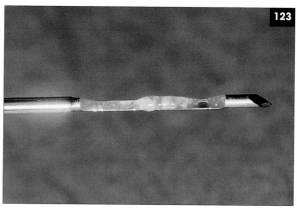

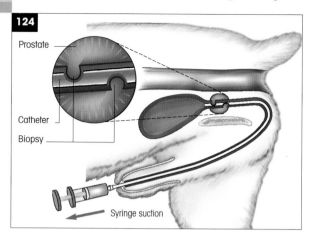

124
Prostate
Catheter
Biopsy
Syringe suction

124 Diagram illustrating the catheter biopsy technique of Melhoff and Osborne (1977). The catheter tip is introduced to the level of the tissues to be biopsied (in this case, the prostatic urethra), as judged from previous clinical and radiographic investigations. A syringe is attached to the catheter and used to apply suction. Pieces of tissue are sucked into the side holes of the catheter and dislodged by moving the catheter to and fro. The catheter is then withdrawn and the pieces of tissue flushed out of the catheter (using formol saline) into a container of formol saline. Experience suggests that it is easier to obtain biopsies from diseased (e.g. neoplastic or inflamed) tissues than from normal urothelium and its surrounding tissues. The small pieces of tissue obtained are aggregated by centrifugation, fixed, sectioned, stained and examined (see **125, 126**). The pieces are not always large enough to allow orientation of the sample by a veterinary pathologist, but this is often not essential. In most cases the differentiation of neoplastic from inflammatory tissue is sufficient for diagnostic purposes. Tiny fragments may be treated as cytology samples and smeared on a slide to be examined microscopically.

125, 126 Histological appearance of material obtained from a catheter biopsy: H&E x100 (**125**) and x300 (**126**). This catheter biopsy was from a nine-year-old castrated male German Shepherd Dog with a prostatic urethral carcinoma.

Problems

THE MAIN PROBLEMS with needle biopsy techniques are haemorrhage from or into the organ biopsied and iatrogenic trauma to this or adjacent organs (**127, 128**). In addition, attempts to biopsy infected (especially abscessed) organs may result in dissemination of infection. The risk of introducing infection with the biopsy needle itself can be minimized by careful attention to sterile technique.

The catheter biopsy technique shares the problems associated with urethral catheterization described previously, but otherwise is free of complications.

127, 128 (**127**) Postmortem appearance of a feline kidney, one week after a Tru-cut biopsy. Note the pale areas associated with renal infarction.
(**128**) A section through the kidney demonstrates that the biopsy needle had been introduced too deep, damaging the renal arcuate vessels at the corticomedullary junction and leading to thrombosis and infarction.

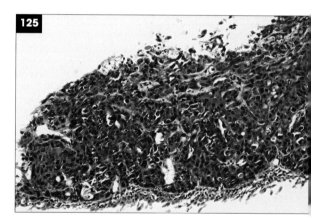

125

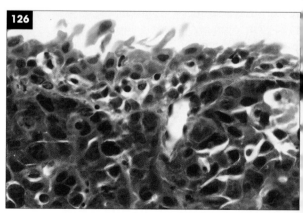

126

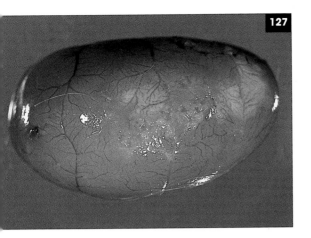

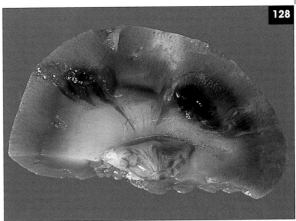

Blood and urine analyses

Indications

HAEMATOLOGICAL AND BIOCHEMICAL examination of blood are indicated in animals with dysuria or haematuria. They are of less value in incontinent animals (unless the animal's incontinence is related to polydipsia/polyuria). Haematology is mainly of use in assessing the degree of anaemia (in animals with severe haematuria or renal disease), dehydration (for example, the vomiting dysuric patient) and toxaemia/bacteraemia (e.g. acute prostatitis or prostatic abscessation). Biochemistry can be used to evaluate the degree of pre-renal, renal or post-renal azotaemia in dysuric animals, but it is also valuable in assessing renal function before nephrectomy or nephrotomy is performed. In cases of suspected bladder rupture, comparison of blood and ascitic fluid creatinine levels is a useful diagnostic aid. If uroperitoneum is present, ascitic fluid levels of creatinine will be markedly higher than those in the blood (comparisons of urea levels are less reliable, since urea diffuses readily across the peritoneum and thus blood and peritoneal fluid levels tend to equilibrate).

Urine biochemistry may provide further information on the nature and degree of renal damage, but it is mainly of value (along with urine cytology) in detecting the presence of microscopic haematuria. Urine bacteriology is mandatory in most animals with urological signs; even if urinary tract infections are not the main cause of the clinical signs, they are frequently present as secondary complications and, if possible, should be eliminated before urological surgery is carried out. This is particularly true in animals in which ureteral transplantation is to be performed (see Chapter 8, p. 134). Dogs with prostatic infections frequently shed organisms into the urine and, therefore, urine bacteriology is valuable in such cases, particularly if it is not possible to sample prostatic secretions or abscesses directly.

A guide to normal values

THERE IS A VAST ARRAY of commercial laboratories offering a service for the analysis of veterinary samples, although the increasing availability of desk top analysers means that even those practices without practice laboratories are now performing routine laboratory examinations. The analytical techniques required vary between analysers and laboratories and will not be described here. A few basic principles are worth mentioning, however.

It is important to know the range of normal values for the variables being assessed for that particular laboratory or analyser. Most commercial laboratories will supply details of their 'normal' values, as may the manufacturers of some analysers. However, in the latter instance, experience with the use of the analyser will lead to a knowledge of the ranges of normality that can be expected. Variations in normality should also be considered. For example, young animals often have a lymphocytosis and lower packed cell volume (PCV) and haemoglobin levels: fit, working dogs (e.g. Greyhounds, Whippets) normally have PCVs that would be considered high for other dogs.

Table 8 Normal biochemical ranges

Analyte	Units	Dog	Cat
Albumin	g/l	32–38	24–35
Globulin	g/l	20–35	21–51
A:G ratio		0.6–1.5	0.4–1.3
ALT	u/l	20–60	15–45
Ammonia	µmol/l	0–50	0–50
Amylase	u/l	450–1,000	450–1,000
Lipase	u/l	0–300	0–300
AST	u/l	20–35	0–20
Bile acids	µmol/l	0–20	0–20
Calcium	mmol/l	2.3–2.6	2.3–2.5
Cholesterol	mmol/l	3.5–7.0	4.0–10.0
Triglycerides	mmol/l	0–1.0	0–1.0
CK	u/l	75–230	50–150
Creatinine	µmol/l	70–110	110–160
Glucose	mmol/l	3.5–5.0	3.5–5.5
Phosphate	mmol/l	0.75–1.25	0.95–1.55
LDH	u/l	35–450	130–470
Lipase	u/l	0–300	0–300
Magnesium	mmol/l	0.8–1.1	0.8–1.1
Potassium	mmol/l	3.5–4.5	4.0–5.0
ALP	u/l	0–110	15–60
Sodium	mmol/l	135–150	149–157
Total bilirubin	µmol/l	0–10	0–10
Total proteins	g/l	63–71	77–91
Urea	mmol/l	2.0–7.0	6.5–10.5

Table 9 Normal haematological values

Estimation	Units	Dog	Cat
PCV	l/l	0.35–0.45	0.25–0.48
RBCs	$\times 10^{12}$/l	5.4–8.0	5.5–10.0
Haemoglobin	g/l	120–180	80–150
MCH	pg	22.0–25.0	12.5–17.0
MCHC	g/l	350–370	300–350
MCV	fl	65.0–75.0	40.0–55.0
Platelets	$\times 10^9$/l	170–500	200–700
WBCs	$\times 10^9$/l	5.5–17.0	4.9–19.0
Differential WBC counts			
Neutrophils	$\times 10^9$/l	3.0–11.5	2.4–12.5
Lymphocytes	$\times 10^9$/l	0.7–3.6	1.4–6.0
Monocytes	$\times 10^9$/l	0.1–1.5	0.1–0.7
Eosinophils	$\times 10^9$/l	0.2–1.4	0.1–1.6
Basophils	$\times 10^9$/l	0–0.1	0–0.1

Table 10 Normal urinalysis values

Estimation	Dog	Cat
pH	5.0–7.0	5.0–7.0
Specific gravity	1.015–1.045	1.015–1.060
Protein	negative	negative
Blood	negative	negative
Haemoglobin	negative	negative
Glucose	negative	negative
Ketones	negative	negative
Bilirubin	negative/trace	negative/trace
Urobilinogen	negative	negative
Urine production	24–40 ml/kg/day	22–30 ml/kg/day

The reference ranges of normal values used in the clinical laboratories at the Bristol Veterinary School are given as a guide (*Tables 8–10*).

Problems

IF BLOOD AND URINE SAMPLES are to be posted, they should be prepared and packed in an appropriate way. Most laboratories prefer blood to be clotted and the serum decanted and submitted for analysis rather than whole blood. Apart from the obvious problem that the sample may haemolyse, serum levels of potassium in whole blood tend to increase during transit (as potassium leaks from blood cells). This may lead to a misdiagnosis of hyperkalaemia and inappropriate therapy.

If urine is posted to a laboratory for bacteriological culture, there may be overgrowth of organisms of low pathogenicity during transit, masking the significant bacteria. This can be prevented by placing the fresh urine sample in a receptacle containing boric acid powder in the proportion of 20 ml of urine to 200 mg of boric acid powder. There is increasing evidence that urine bacteriology should be quantitative as well as qualitative and that low counts of bacteria are of no clinical significance. Opinions vary on what is meant by 'low counts', but in general, if a sample is obtained by aseptic catheterization, counts of <1,000 and <100 organisms per ml are taken to be due to contamination in dogs and cats, respectively. If the sample is taken by cystocentesis, this figure is <100 organisms per ml in both species.

If samples are posted to a commercial laboratory, it is a legal obligation that the post office guidelines are followed for their package and labelling. Apart from the illegality of inadequate packing and labelling and the health hazards to handlers, urine and blood samples squeezed from sodden envelopes are of little diagnostic value.

Urodynamics

Indications

SUSPECTED ABNORMAL FUNCTIONING of the lower urinary tract such as urethral sphincter mechanism incompetence, detrusor instability, reflex dyssynergia and neurogenic abnormalities.

Techniques

TECHNIQUES INCLUDED within urodynamics are:

* Urethral pressure profilometry ('resting' or 'stressed').
* Cystometry.
* Electromyography.

In small animal practice, most work has been done on resting urethral pressure profilometry and indications for other urodynamic techniques are uncommon. However, all of these techniques are subject to a wide variety of artefacts and variations in the results obtained. Apart from the fact that they are not available in most veterinary practices (and unlikely to be so in the foreseeable future), they have proved to be of less diagnostic value than was first hoped. Therefore, a brief description only will be given of urethral pressure profilometry (**129, 130**). There is additional information in the Further Reading section at the end of this book.

129 During urethral pressure profilometry, a catheter with a pressure-measuring device at or near the tip is inserted into the bladder and then withdrawn along the urethra (**a**). The pressure can be measured by the resistance to outflow of fluid from catheter side holes (perfusion profilometry), pressure changes within balloons or using microtip pressure transducers. The latter are preferable but are expensive. As the catheter passes along the urethra, a graph of pressure against distance is produced on a recorder: this is the resting urethral pressure profile (**b**). A number of variables, defined by the International Continence Society, can be measured from the graph.

130 Subtracted urethral pressure profile recordings from a continent bitch (**a**) and an incontinent bitch (**b**). A 'subtracted' profile makes allowances for variations in intravesical pressure such as those due to respiration (regular small peaks). Subtracted profilometry involves the simultaneous measurement of intra-urethral and intravesical pressures. The intravesical pressure is continuously subtracted from the intra-urethral pressure to give a more accurate representation of the urodynamic event, the subtracted urethral pressure profile. This is summarized in **a**, but **b** shows only the subtracted profile. The profile from the

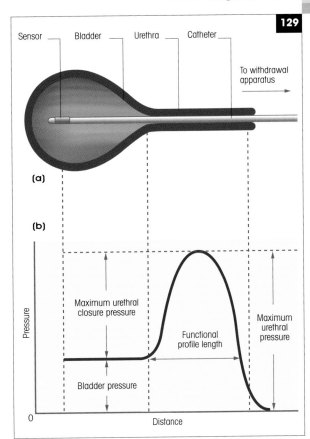

129

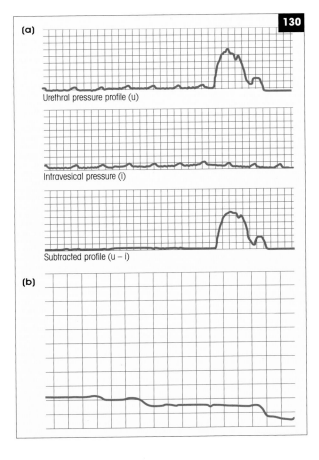

130

continent animal conforms to the previous diagram (**129**), but urethral resistance in the incontinent bitch is less than intravesical pressure throughout the profile. It would be nice if all profiles were as diagnostic of good or poor urethral function as these two examples, but, unfortunately, this is not the case.

Problems

IN ORDER TO MINIMIZE VARIATIONS, it is imperative that a standard technique is used. Following study of variables such as the position of the animal, orientation of the catheter within the urethra, method of chemical restraint, size of catheter, catheter material, catheter withdrawal rate and degree of bladder filling, the following standards have been suggested:

- The animal should be positioned in right lateral recumbency.
- The catheter should be orientated so that the side hole (if a perfusion technique is used) or microtip transducer is facing dorsally within the urethra.
- The catheter should be as narrow and soft as possible; in practice, this usually means a 3–4Fr polyurethane catheter in cats and a 6–8Fr silicone rubber catheter in dogs. Softer catheters are available, but they are more difficult to insert and, if microtip catheters are used, more liable to damage.
- A standard method of chemical restraint should be used in all cases. However, a perfect anaesthetic or relaxant (i.e. one that has no effect on the urodynamic variables being measured) has yet to be discovered.
- The catheter should be withdrawn at a speed of 1 mm/second or less.
- The bladder should be filled with sterile saline or emptied of urine to achieve a resting intravesical pressure of 5 cm H_2O.

Once the method has been standardized, it is important to determine the range of normality using that method, since this will vary from centre to centre. Meaningful conclusions can only be drawn when normal values are known.

Belt driven catheter withdrawal devices are unsuitable, since they do not prevent the weight of the catheter or its lead from pulling the catheter from the urethra. It is preferable to use a rod driven device, which clips directly on to the catheter (**131**).

The use of a single sensor on the catheter makes the assumption that intravesical pressure remains constant as the sensor passes along the urethra. This problem can be overcome by the use of two sensors – 'simultaneous' urethral pressure profilometry (**130–132**).

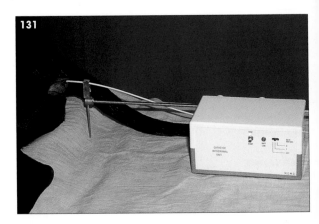

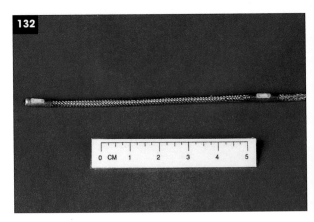

131 The problems of inadvertent pulling of the catheter from the urethra and catheter rotation are overcome by the use of a rod driven device that clips directly onto the catheter.

132 Double sensor catheter used to measure (simultaneously) intravesical and urethral pressures. The microtip transducer at the tip of this silicone rubber catheter remains in the bladder throughout profilometry, while the second sensor starts in the bladder but then passes along the urethra during withdrawal. An electronic subtraction unit in the recorder continuously subtracts the intravesical pressure from the urethral pressure, resulting in a more accurate 'subtracted' pressure profile (see **130**). In most animals in which urethral pressure profilometry is indicated (i.e. incontinent large breeds of female dog with suspected urethral sphincter mechanism incompetence), the tip and second sensors should be separated by 8 cm to allow the tip sensor to remain in the bladder throughout profilometry.

Endoscopy

Indications

ALTHOUGH LAPAROSCOPY can be applied to small animal urological cases, the most commonly used endoscopic technique is urethrocystoscopy (**133, 134**). The indications, therefore, are suspected lesions of the bladder or urethra. In humans, surgical procedures (e.g. transurethral prostatic resection) can be performed endoscopically. Unfortunately, the smaller size of the canine urethra means that endoscopic procedures are usually limited to obtaining biopsy material (unless the endoscope is inserted via a cystotomy), since the diameters of resectoscopes are usually too great to permit introduction into the urethras of small animals. Smaller, paediatric resectoscopes are becoming available, which may allow resection techniques in small animals in the future.

The main advantage of urethrocystoscopy is the ability to visualize, and thus take an accurate biopsy from, urethral or bladder lesions. If lithotrypsy equipment is available, endoscopic fragmentation of vesical calculi can be performed. The cystoscope can also be used to guide catheters into the ureters, thus allowing sampling of urine from individual kidneys (e.g. in suspected cases of idiopathic renal haemorrhage) as a less traumatic alternative to cystotomy.

Techniques

A VARIETY OF EQUIPMENT is available and most is designed for use in humans rather than animals. It is also rather expensive. Urethrocystoscopy technique will not be described in this book; rather, the reader is referred to the more extensive descriptions of the apparatus available and its use in the sections on urethrocystoscopy by Brearley *et al* (1991), Senior (1999) and McCarthy (2005).

Problems

URETHROCYSTOSCOPY is associated with the same potential problems as introduction of other instruments into the lower urinary tract (see Urethral catheterization, p. 38) and is contraindicated in the presence of acute bacterial infections, which it may exacerbate.

133 Urethroscopic appearance of a urethral carcinoma in a bitch. This bitch was dysuric and the urethra can be seen to be almost completely occluded by abnormal, white, vascular tissue. This lesion was readily detectable on retrograde positive contrast vagino-urethrography and the diagnosis was confirmed by means of a catheter biopsy.

134 Urethrocystoscopy does allow more accurate collection of biopsy material if the lesion is more discreet, as in this case of localized, diphtheritic cystitis. In this German Shepherd Dog bitch, double contrast cystography had revealed a proliferative lesion near the bladder neck ('skylined' in this illustration). It would have been difficult to obtain an accurate biopsy using the catheter biopsy technique in this case.

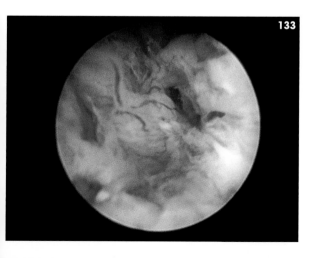

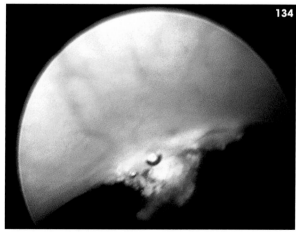

DIFFERENTIAL DIAGNOSIS AND TREATMENT

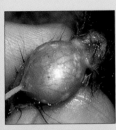

4 Non-prostatic dysuria

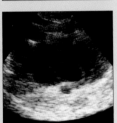

5 Prostatic disorders

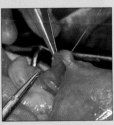

6 Urinary tract trauma

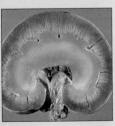

7 Other causes of haematuria

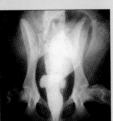

8 Urinary incontinence

4 Non-prostatic dysuria

A stream ran small and terrible and shrill; it was so still;
Hilda Doolittle (1886–1961)

FOR THE PURPOSES OF THIS SECTION, dysuria is defined as difficulty in urination. The differential diagnosis of dysuria in the dog is:

- Urethral calculus.
- Prostatic disorders (see Chapter 5).
- Bladder neck neoplasia.
- Urethral neoplasia.
- Urethral trauma (see Chapter 6).
- Urethritis.
- Urethral stricture (see Chapter 6).

- Neurogenic dysuria (upper or lower motor neurone lesions).
- Bladder displacement/entrapment.
- Functional disorders (e.g. dyssynergia, bladder atony).
- 'External' resistance to urine outflow (e.g. ureterocoele [rarely]).

In the cat, dysuria other than that associated with FUS/FLUTD is rare.

Diagnosis

A DIAGNOSIS often has to wait. In cases of complete urinary retention, the bladder must be emptied by catheterization (see **89–101**) or centesis (see **112**) to prevent secondary vesical problems. There are a number of experimental papers detailing the effects of obstruction on the bladder and some are listed in the Further Reading section at the end of this book. Clinically recognizable problems include urothelial sloughing, deeper ischaemic damage and paralysis (see **2** and **135**). The metabolic effects of uraemia, acidosis and hyperkalaemia should be corrected using intravenous fluids, bladder drainage and, if uroperitoneum is present, abdominocentesis and peritoneal dialysis (see **113, 114**). There is some argument about the use of intravenous Hartmann's solution (compound sodium lactate) in such cases. Although Hartmann's solution contains potassium, and thus might be expected to make the hyperkalaemia worse, it also tends to correct the acidosis. The author's approach is to use fluids without potassium initially (normal saline or dextrose saline) and then, once the potassium levels enter the upper end of the normal range, to change to Hartmann's, since many animals that were initially hyperkalaemic may become hypokalaemic as acid-base balance is restored. If the animal is severely acidotic, bicarbonate can be added to the initial fluids.

Once the animal's condition is stabilized, a diagnosis can be attempted. The examination should include the above catheterization plus detailed clinical, radiographic and laboratory techniques (see Part 1).

135 Effects of ischaemia on the bladder. Dysuria recurred in this cat one week after relief of a urethral obstruction. On the second occasion the bladder neck became obstructed by necrotic urothelium secondary to bladder wall ischaemia. The dead tissue had sloughed into the bladder lumen and is shown during the cystotomy to remove it.

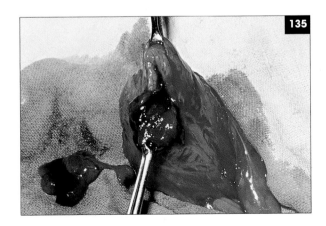

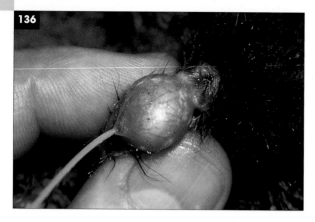

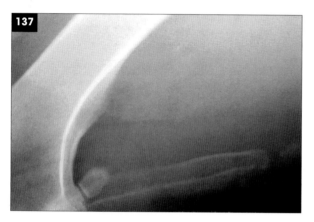

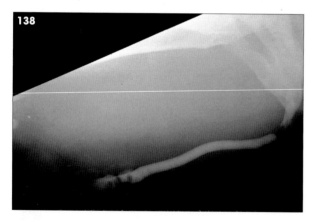

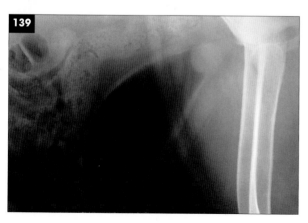

In some animals the lesion may be palpable (e.g. bladder neck or urethral masses and calculi) or even visible (**136**). The most useful radiographic technique is retrograde positive contrast urethrocystography or vagino-urethrography, which will demonstrate most urethral (and some prostatic) conditions including non-radiopaque calculi. The extra time taken performing contrast radiography is often well spent (**137, 138**). Subsequent introduction of air into the bladder will result in a double contrast cystogram, useful in the diagnosis of bladder neck neoplasia and bladder displacement (see **75, 76, 78, 79**). Occasionally, bladder neck tumours will show up on pneumocystography alone (**139**), but double contrast cystography is better.

Differentiation of urethral tumours from urethritis may be difficult (**140**), but biopsy via a catheter is a valuable, non-invasive diagnostic aid (see **124–126**).

Bladder neck tumours are usually urothelial in origin and are frequently malignant carcinomas (see **78, 79**). However, in young, large breeds of dogs malignant bladder rhabdomyosarcomas may occur, albeit rarely (**141**). There are occasional reports of their successful removal, but all cases seen by the author have been inoperable. Benign tumours are papillomas, polyps and leiomyomas (**139, 142–144**).

136 The calcium carbonate calculus causing the penile urethral obstruction in this rabbit is obvious and was removed via a urethrotomy. The rabbit subsequently underwent a cystotomy to remove a vesical calculus that was also present.

137, 138 Plain radiograph (**137**) and retrograde positive contrast urethrogram (**138**) of the penile urethra of a dysuric German Shepherd Dog. The osseous reaction at the caudal end of the os penis seen on the plain radiograph is not calculus material; the calculi can be seen outlined by contrast medium on the urethrogram. The urethrogram also illustrates a urethral stricture just ventral to the ischium (possibly due to attempts to push the calculi back into the bladder using a catheter). This stricture would have been missed if urethrography had not been performed.

139 A bladder neck tumour (leiomyoma) demonstrated by pneumocystography. This tumour was acting as a ball valve at the bladder neck, resulting in intermittent dysuria. A catheter was passed easily in this dog and failed to indicate any obstruction. This tumour was excised by suburothelial resection via a cystotomy.

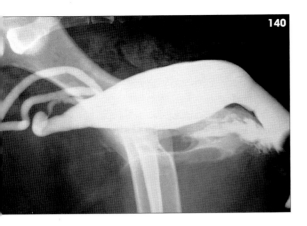

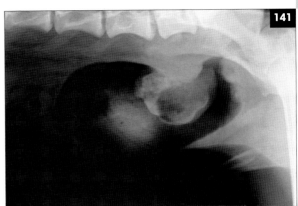

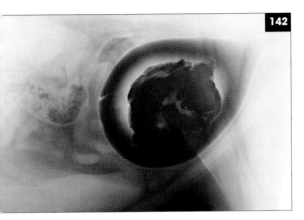

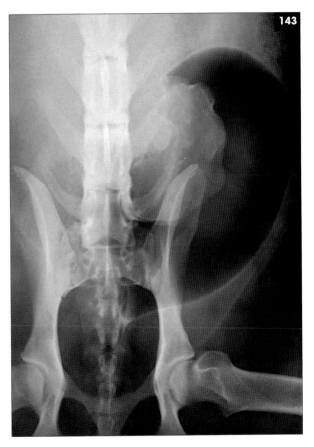

140 Chronic urethritis in an adult Rough Collie bitch demonstrated by retrograde positive contrast vagino-urethrography. Note the similarity in radiographic appearance to urethral cancer (see **52**). A catheter biopsy technique (see **124–126**) is a useful way of differentiating these conditions.

141 Rhabdomyosarcoma of the dorsal bladder wall and bladder neck demonstrated by double contrast cystography in a male one-year-old Doberman Pinscher.

142–144 The large mass demonstrated by lateral (**142**) and ventrodorsal (**143**) double contrast cystography in this dog proved to be a benign polyp, which was exteriorized via a cystotomy (**144**) and excised across its pedicle. Such polyps appear to be associated with chronic irritation (e.g. chronic infections or uroliths). However, in many cases the exact predisposing cause cannot be determined and the masses may recur. It is worth culturing excised tissue (as well as urine) in addition to submitting it for histopathology. Sometimes, organisms can be detected in the polyp tissue but not in the urine, and appropriate antibiotic therapy can be instituted. This may be a form of interstitial cystitis.

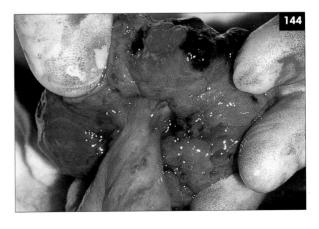

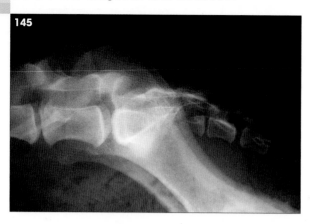

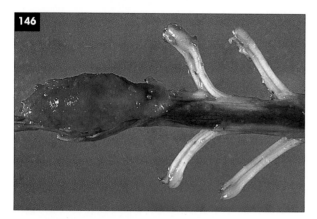

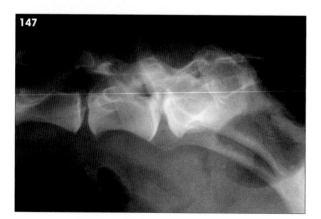

Neurogenic dysuria associated with an upper motor neurone (UMN) lesion (e.g. thoracolumbar disc disease) is due to lack of higher control of the micturition reflex, whereas in cases of a lower motor neurone (LMN) lesion, the pathways of the reflex itself are affected. Without MRI or CT scanning, LMN lesions can be difficult to diagnose unless other signs of cauda equina disease are present (145–148). A form of LMN dysuria may follow obstructive dysuria after the obstruction is relieved. This is presumably due to bladder wall stretching, inflammation and reduced perfusion, leading to bladder wall ischaemia, breakdown of tight junctions and reduced neuromuscular function.

145–147 Examples of LMN disorders leading to dysuria (urinary retention with overflow incontinence); all of these dogs walked into the consulting room.
(**145**) Fracture of the caudal sacrum of a German Shepherd Dog after a road traffic accident. Sacral fractures and sacrococcygeal injuries are more common in cats.
(**146**) Extradural osteosarcoma of the cauda equina seen post mortem in a cross-bred dog. On initial presentation, this dog showed no neurological deficits apart from loss of bladder function and dysuria. Three weeks later, the animal began to carry the tail to one side. A myelogram at that time was suspicious of a cauda equina lesion and the dog was euthanased.
(**147**) Lumbosacral disc prolapse in a great Dane. The diagnosis in all of these cases would have been greatly facilitated by more sophisticated imaging modalities such as MRI scanning.

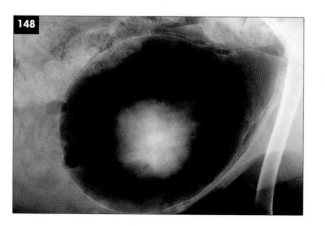

148 In animals with urinary retention, urinary tract infection is more likely. Although double contrast cystography has been performed in this English Setter with neurogenic dysuria, the air within the bladder wall tissues is due to the presence of gas-producing organisms; this dog has secondary emphysematous cystitis.

Treatment

ONCE THE ANIMAL IS STABILIZED, treatment can be
carried out. In dogs with urethral calculi it should be
borne in mind that bladder stones are usually also
present. Urethrotomy should be a last resort because of
the risks of complications (see below). It is safer to
return any urethral calculi to the bladder using
the technique of retrograde hydropropulsion (**149**) and
then to remove all stones via a cystotomy (**150–160**).

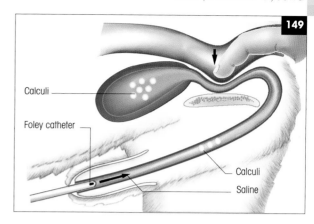

149 Diagram illustrating retrograde hydropropulsion
of urethral calculi (after Piermattei and Osborne,
1977). The bladder is emptied by cystocentesis.
A gloved finger is inserted *per rectum* and used to
compress the pelvic urethra against the pubis. An 8Fr
Foley catheter is inserted into the penile urethra and
its cuff inflated with 2–3 ml of air (alternatively, a
polyurethane catheter can be used and the urethra
occluded around it with digital pressure). Sterile saline
is injected through the catheter. This results in
dilation of the urethra (which can be appreciated
beneath the ball of the finger in the rectum), thus
freeing the calculi from the surrounding urethral wall.
The digital pressure on the pelvic urethra is released
(while saline continues to be injected), allowing the
calculi to be flushed retrogradely into the bladder.
Several attempts may have to be made before all the
urethral calculi are returned to the bladder, and the
success of the technique should be confirmed radiographically. If all the calculi are seen to have been
returned to the bladder on a radiograph, the urethra is
catheterized (to empty the bladder and to prevent
calculi from returning to the urethra) and the animal
taken to theatre for cystotomy to remove the vesical
uroliths (see **150–158**).

150 During cystotomy for removal of calculi,
retrograde flushing should be used to remove calculi
from the bladder neck and proximal urethra. These
are not detectable by palpation. Sterile saline should
be used to flush small stones onto a swab placed
adjacent to the laparotomy wound, as shown.

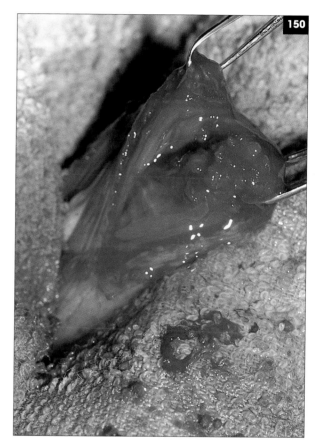

151–153 Diagrams illustrating the author's preferred method of bladder closure. A two-layered closure is used. The first layer is a continuous Czerny suture, shown in a section through the bladder incision (**151**), to appose the bladder wall incisions. The bladder wall is then inverted using Lembert (**152**) or Cushing (**153**) suture patterns (the Cushing suture pattern is illustrated on an external view of the bladder incision). If the bladder wall is grossly thickened, inversion may not be possible and one may have to rely on appositional closure alone. If simple interrupted sutures are used, the bladder should be filled with sterile saline after closure to confirm that no leakage occurs between sutures.

154–160 Closure of the bladder using continuous Czerny followed by continuous Cushing suture patterns. All sutures begin and end beyond the ends of the bladder wall incision. The author prefers to use synthetic absorbable suture material, which should be swaged on to the needle.

(**154**) The Czerny suture is begun by taking a bite through the bladder wall (but not into the lumen) just beyond one end of the incision. After tying the knot, the short end of the suture is not cut, but is grasped with clamps. This can then be used to support that part of the bladder and to provide something to pull against as the suture is tightened.

(**155**) The Czerny suture is used to appose the edges of the wound without passing through the urothelium (i.e. the suture is taken through the bladder serosa and detrusor muscle down to the suburothelium only). The suturing continues from left to right (in this Figure) to beyond the right hand end of the incision and is then tied. The suture is left attached to the right hand end knot and an inverting suture placed in a continuous fashion from right to left.

(**156**) Here, a continuous Cushing pattern is being used. The suture is taken in and out of the bladder wall adjacent to the far side of the incision and parallel to it without entering the bladder lumen.

(**157**) The suture is then taken into the bladder wall on the near side of the incision (see **153**). Again, it is passed through the bladder wall parallel to the incision.

(**158**) To illustrate the inversion effect of the Cushing suture, a number of bites of suture have been placed but not tightened. The Czerny sutures are still visible.

(**159**) When the suture is tightened, the bladder wall is inverted, thus burying the layer of Czerny sutures.

(**160**) When the inverting layer has been completed, the suture can either be tied to itself or to the short end of the suture material that remained attached to the initial knot of the Czerny suture.

151

Bladder urothelium

Bladder seromuscular layer

152

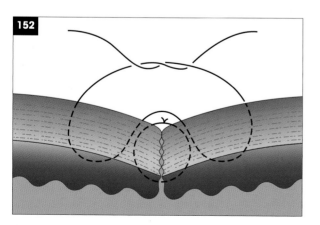

153

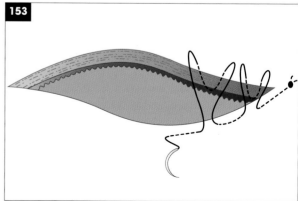

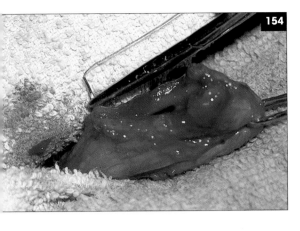

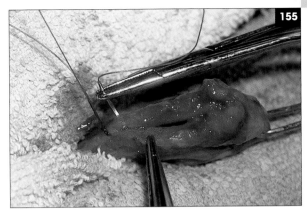

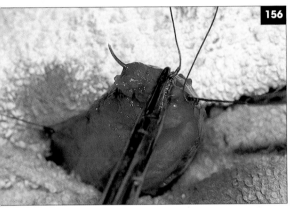

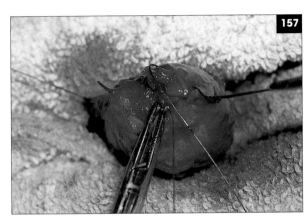

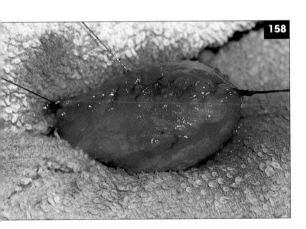

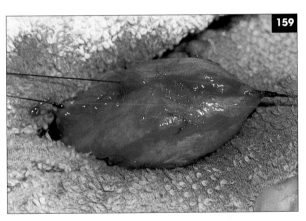

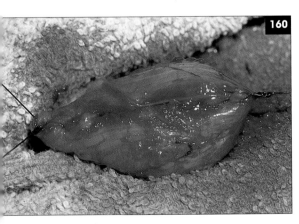

If retrograde hydropropulsion is not successful, urethral calculi should be removed via a urethrotomy (161–166) and the vesical calculi removed later when the urethrotomy has healed. Urethrotomy and cystotomy should not be performed simultaneously; if the urethrotomy becomes obstructed with blood clots, the increased intravesical pressure may lead to cystotomy breakdown and/or leakage of urine into the peritoneum. Complications after urethrotomy include:

- Haemorrhage. Bleeding from the wound is usually stimulated by urination or overexcitement and can last up to ten days.
- Infiltration of ventral abdominal tissues with urine. Related to malalignment of skin and urethral incisions. Associated with urine scalding and possibly occlusion of the skin incision. May need further surgery to create a larger opening. If the scrotum becomes infiltrated with urine, scrotal necrosis may occur and castration with scrotal ablation (see 288–294) may be required.
- Blood clots. May obstruct the urethra. Clear using a catheter.
- Non healing. A permanent urethral fistula results (rare). Remedy by suturing.
- Scar tissue formation. Postsurgical and/or calculus trauma. May lead to stricture (167). A more proximal urethrostomy may be needed to bypass the stricture (see 187–199 and 352–355).
- Rarely, a urethral diverticulum can develop at the site of a urethrotomy (168).

161–166 (**161**) The commonest site for urethrotomy is at the caudal end of the os penis, since this is the most likely location of urethral calculi. The incision should not be too close to the scrotum; this reduces the risk of urine tracking subcutaneously into the scrotum, resulting in scrotal necrosis.
(**162**) The retractor penis muscle (which is somewhat vestigial in the dog compared with ruminants) is identified. It can be incised in the midline or retracted to one side to allow access to the penis.
(**163**) In this case the retractor penis muscle is being held aside with forceps and the penis lifted. This allows the ventral groove of the os penis to be seen (or palpated) and used as a guide for a midline incision.
(**164**) The penis is incised in the midline. Textbooks often describe an avascular median raphe, but this is rarely located during surgery. The incision should pass between the corpora spongiosa and through the ventral urethral urothelium into the urethral lumen, as shown. Once the penis is no longer lifted, haemorrhage usually occurs from the corpora spongiosa. This can be controlled by direct pressure. In the author's experience, local adrenaline has little, if any, effect on the haemorrhage.
(**165, 166**) The calculi are removed from the urethra using alligator forceps. Urethral patency is then confirmed by passage of a urinary catheter distally and proximally from the urethrotomy incision.
The urethrotomy incision is left open to heal by secondary intention and the owners warned to expect haemorrhage, particularly after the dog urinates. The wound usually heals within 5–7 days.

167 Repeated urethrotomies for recurring urolithiasis in this German Shepherd Dog have resulted in urethral stricture. The retrograde positive contrast urethrogram demonstrates the severe disruption of normal urethral anatomy. This case underlines two points: urethrotomy should be avoided if possible and any calculi obtained should be analysed so that suitable prophylactic measures can be instituted and the possibility of recurrence minimized.

168 A urethral diverticulum containing over 30 calculi in a Basset Hound. The diverticulum resulted from closure of a previous urethrotomy skin incision (in an attempt to control postoperative haemorrhage) and subsequent outgrowth of urethral urothelium into the subcutaneous space to form a pouch. As further calculi from the bladder travelled down the urethra, they passed into the pouch, which, when full, resulted in compression of the urethra and further dysuria. The pouch and calculi had to be excised.

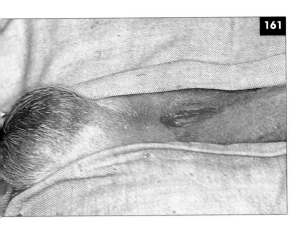

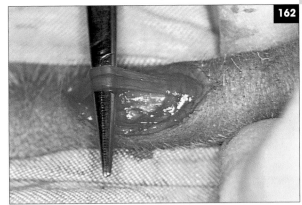

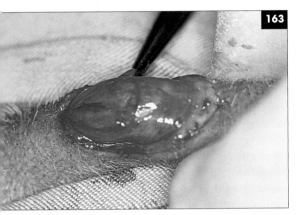

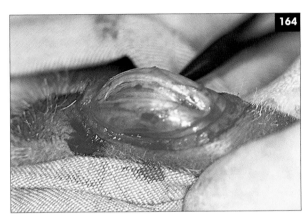

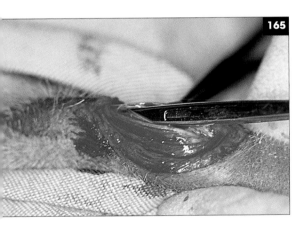

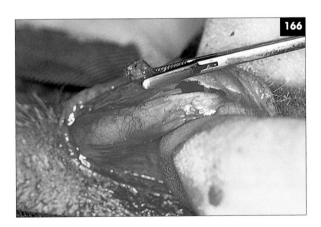

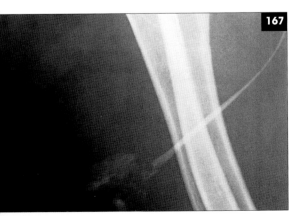

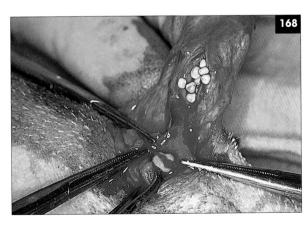

In male cats with urolithiasis, discrete calculi may be returned to the bladder by retrograde flushing and removed as described for the dog (see above). In the case of sabulous obstruction of the urethra, the crystals are flushed retrogradely into the bladder (see **100–103**) and then removed by bladder lavage using a catheter or dissolution *in situ* after their nature has been identified. The sabulous material obstructing the urethra may prevent adequate insertion of a cat catheter to allow flushing (because of the side holes). In such patients, lacrimal cannulae are useful (see **100–103**).

The author prefers sterile normal saline as a flushing solution. Once the obstruction is relieved, an indwelling catheter is inserted (and the cat fitted with an Elizabethan collar) to allow the animal and its bladder to recover from the effects of the obstruction. The catheter is left *in situ* for 3–4 days. In some cats urethral obstruction and the resulting increase in intravesical pressure open up congenital vesico-urachal diverticula, which may be detected during contrast radiography or ultrasonography. These rarely require surgical treatment; they usually resolve spontaneously after the obstruction is relieved.

In cats which repeatedly obstruct and/or develop penile urethral strictures (**169, 170**), perineal urethrostomy may be required, but preferably this should be done as an elective rather than emergency procedure (**169–181**).

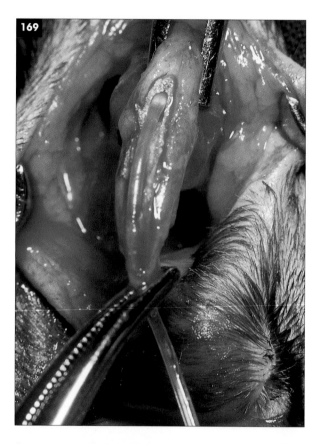

169, 170 (**169**) The worst time to have to perform a feline perineal urethrostomy. This cat's urethra was so impacted with crystals that attempts at retrograde flushing failed. A catheter could not be passed until the urethra was incised during an emergency perineal urethrostomy. The presence of the sabulous uroliths causes secondary urethritis, making tissue identification more difficult. In addition, the friable tissues do not hold sutures very well.
(**170**) Priapism is another indication for perineal urethrostomy in the cat; ultimately, drying of the penis results in stricture of the external urethral orifice.

171–179 Perineal urethrostomy in the cat is performed with the animal in the same position as for the dog. The operation is best done as an elective procedure rather than at the time of urethral obstruction. Apart from allowing the cat to recover from the systemic and local effects of urethral obstruction, this also means that a feline 3Fr or 4Fr urethral catheter can be inserted to facilitate identification of the urethral lumen and to empty the bladder of urine (**171**). If a catheter cannot be passed, the bladder must be emtied by cystocentesis, since a full urinary bladder makes surgery very difficult (its weight tends to pull the membranous urethra cranially). The anus is closed with a purse-string suture.

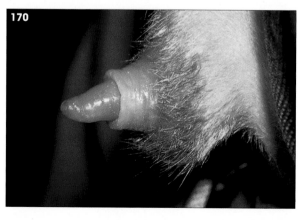

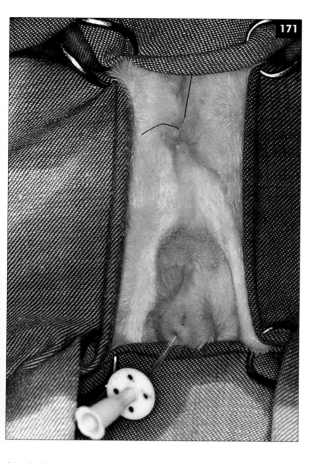

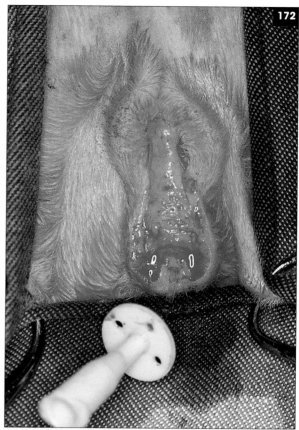

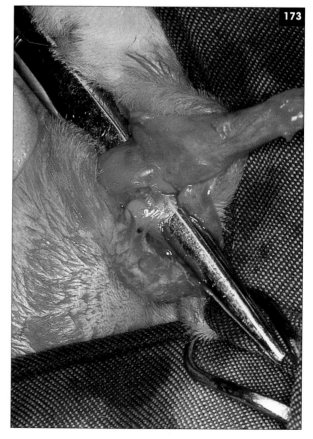

(172) A vertical skin incision is made from just dorsal to the scrotum to the preputial tip. If the animal is entire, it is castrated. If excessive scrotal skin remains, this is excised elliptically. The incision is continued ventrally around the tip of the penis, leaving a small amount of preputial mucosa attached to the ventral part of the skin.

(173) The penis is freed from surrounding fat and fascia by blunt and sharp dissection and the ischiocavernosus muscles identified. In the photograph, Metzenbaum scissors have been placed behind the cat's left ischiocavernosus muscle. Each ischiocavernosus muscle is sectioned at its origin on the tuber ischium; haemorrhage is usually minimal and can be controlled with direct local pressure.

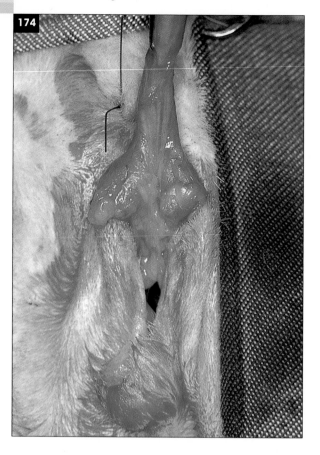

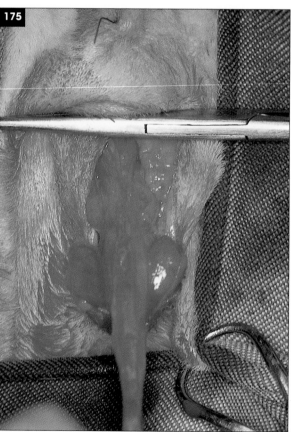

(174) The penis has been reflected dorsally to demonstrate the two, sectioned ischiocavernosus muscles. The ventral fascial attachments of the penis and urethra to the pelvis are broken down by blunt and sharp dissection to allow mobilization of the urethra in a caudal direction. This is virtually impossible if the bladder is full, hence the need to empty the bladder of urine pre-operatively.

(175) The penis and pelvic urethra are freed until the paired bulbo-urethral glands can be identified. These can be seen as bilateral bulges on the dorso-lateral urethra, proximal to the attachments of the ischiocavernosus muscles.

(176) At the level of the bulbo-urethral glands, the narrow penile urethra widens into the membranous urethra and so a urethrotomy is performed at or cranial to this site and not caudal to it on the penile urethra. The urethrotomy incision should be as long as possible to allow for the formation of a large stoma

(177) The dorsal urethral wall at the proximal end of the urethrotomy is sutured to the dorsal end of the skin incision to prevent tension on the suture line postoperatively. The urethral urothelium is sutured to the skin on both sides of the stoma. As the urothelium is rather delicate, it is necessary to include a small bite into the corpus spongiosum to prevent the sutures from tearing out. In the past, the author used absorbable sutures to avoid the necessity of suture removal. These irritated some cats, which licked and traumatized the area sufficiently to result in local oedema and partial obstruction of the stoma. Silk was then tried as a suture material (as shown). Although less irritating, it absorbed blood leaking from the stoma postoperatively. The sutures became entangled in blood clots, which made suture identification and removal difficult. The author now prefers to use 3/0 or 4/0 monofilament nylon. This leads to minimal reaction and is easily identified. Simple interrupted sutures are used in all cases.

(178, 179) The penis is now amputated level with the ventral part of the stoma. The urethrostomy is completed by suturing the fascia ventral to the stoma closed from side to side (using synthetic absorbable material) and then folding the ventral edge of the perineal skin incision (with preputial mucosa attached dorsally. The preputial mucosa is sutured to the ventral urothelium of the penile stump. The two small open skin wounds at 4 and 8 o'clock to the stoma are closed with simple interrupted sutures. The purse-string suture is removed from the anus and the catheter removed from the urethra. A large (6Fr) urinary catheter should be easily passable through the stoma and into the bladder after surgery. Skin sutures are removed after ten days, under sedation or general anaesthesia.

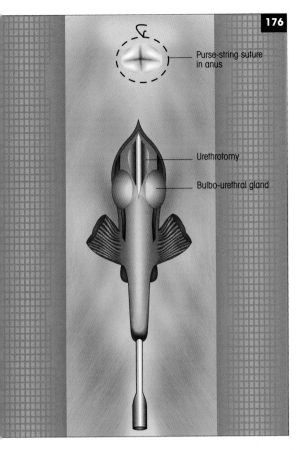

Purse-string suture in anus

Urethrotomy

Bulbo-urethral gland

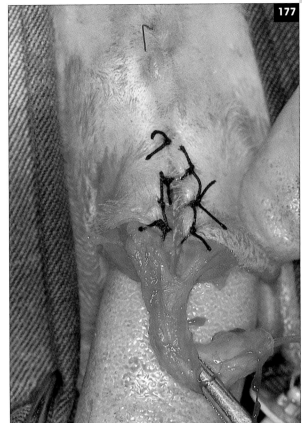

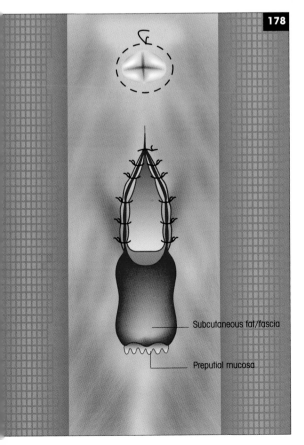

Subcutaneous fat/fascia

Preputial mucosa

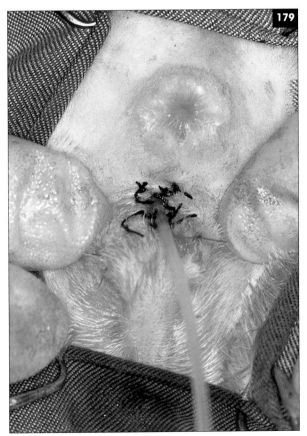

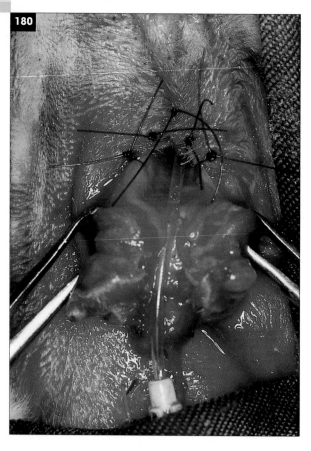

180 Stenosis of the stoma may occur. In this cat the perineal urethrostomy is being revised to excise the stenosed stoma. The urethra has been opened and the narrowing of the urethra can be seen distal to the patent membranous urethra. The stenosis in this case was associated with stomatizing the urethra at an inappropriate site, resulting in a small stoma on a narrow portion of urethra (the stoma was made into the penile urethra rather than the wider membranous urethra). This was corrected by creating a larger stoma into the membranous urethra, as shown, and excising the stenosed penile urethra and previous stoma.

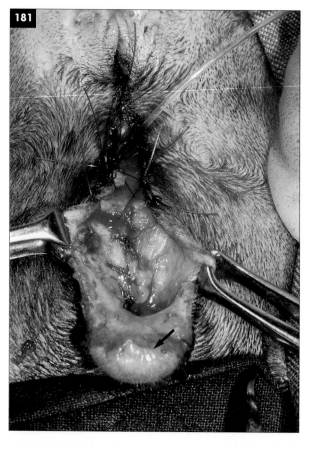

181 Stricture of the stoma is less likely after perineal urethrostomy in cats if the ventral part of the penile urothelium is joined to preputial mucosa rather than preputial skin. In addition, the preputial mucosa ventral to the stoma acts as a 'drainage board' and is less likely to be scalded by urine than skin. In this cat (in which perineal urethrostomy is being performed to relieve urethral stenosis after air gun pellet trauma to the penis), the fascia ventral to the stoma has been closed. The preputial mucosa (arrowed), which was left attached to the prepuce, will be reflected dorsally and attached to the ventral edge of the urethral urothelium to complete the stoma, as described in **179**.

In the case of neurogenic dysuria associated with
intervertebral disc prolapse, mildly affected animals
may respond to conservative treatment, but severe cases
such as those with complete loss of motor, bladder ±
sensory function should be treated as emergencies and
decompressive surgery (fenestration or laminectomy)
performed within 24 hours.

Minor urethral trauma may heal if urinary bypass
is provided using an indwelling urethral or tube cystostomy catheter (see **89, 90** and **231–234**) and conservative treatment, but more extensive urethral ruptures
should be treated surgically. If uroperitoneum
develops, such cases may have the same metabolic
problems as animals with bladder rupture (hyperkalaemia, acidosis and azotaemia) and this must be
corrected before surgical intervention or anaesthesia
or insertion of tube cystostomies. Urethral repair
(especially intrapelvic) is difficult and the exposure is
facilitated by transpubic combined with caudal laparotomy approaches. An indwelling catheter may be
useful as a urethral 'splint' postoperatively. In animals
with gross, irreparable trauma, it is possible to
perform an antepubic urethrostomy, but postoperative scalding of the ventral abdomen with urine and
incontinence may occur and the results are often unacceptable to the owner (see **367–369**). See Chapter 6
(Urinary tract trauma) for further details of urethral
repair, including the treatment of urethral strictures.

Most bladder neck/urethral tumours are malignant
(see **78, 79, 141** and **182, 183**) and only occasionally is
the tumour benign and/or operable (see **139, 142–144**
and **184–199**). In animals with lower urinary tract
malignancy, if the main clinical sign is urinary
frequency/urgency rather than difficulty, some palliation may be obtained with non-steroidal anti-inflam-
matory drugs (NSAIDs), especially cyclooxygenase
inhibitors such as piroxicam or meloxicam. Tube cystostomies, endoscopic or Nd:YAG laser debulking and
urethral stents have also been used to provide palliation
in animals with urethral/prostatic or bladder neck
malignancies.

Urethritis is best treated by means of bypass using
an indwelling urethral or tube cystostomy catheter (see
89, 90 and **231–234**) and parenteral antibiotic therapy
based on bacteriological sensitivities. In some cases,
corticosteroid therapy may also be required. This
condition is termed 'chronic urethritis' because it has a
tendency to recur. The condition can be severe enough
that a urethral caruncle develops and it can be even
more difficult to differentiate from malignancy.

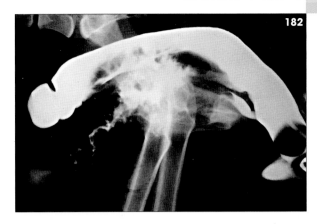

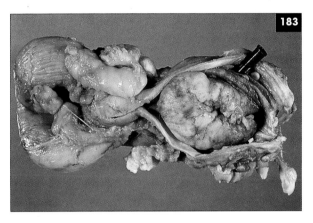

182, 183 Urethral carcinoma demonstrated
by retrograde positive contrast vagino-urethrography
in a cross-bred bitch (**182**). The tumour has
completely obstructed the urethra and the animal can
only urinate (with difficulty) because the tumour has
eroded through the floor of the vagina, seen from
above in the postmortem picture with the vaginal
roof opened (**183**).

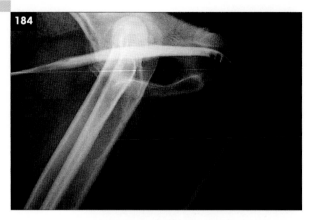

184

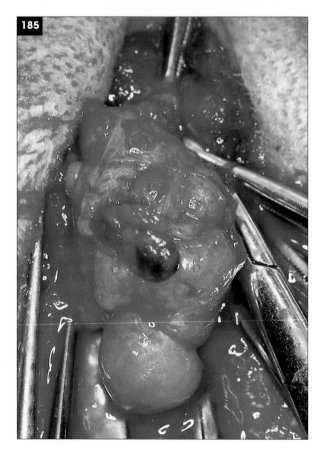

185

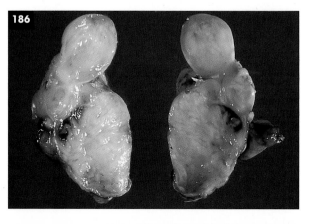

186

184–186 Ischial urethral narrowing in a dysuric male Labrador Retriever demonstrated by retrograde positive contrast urethrography (**184**). This was due to an intramural leiomyosarcoma, which was excised via the perineum (**185**). The excised (sectioned) tumour is shown in **186**. Although leiomyosarcomas are malignant, they are slow to metastasize and this dog was alive and well with no recurrence of signs four years after surgery.

187–199 This adult German Shepherd Dog has a chondrosarcoma of the caudal os penis (**187**). Although malignant, these tumours are slow to metastasize. No metastases were detected and the tumour was excised by penile ablation and scrotal urethrostomy.

(**188**) An eliptical skin incision is made around the penis and scrotum. The branches of the caudal superficial epigastric and external pudendal vessels, which supply the prepuce and scrotum, are identified clamped and ligated along with other subcutaneous vessels.

(**189**) The penis is freed from subcutaneous fat and fascia by a combination of blunt and sharp dissection and is elevated.

(**190**) As the penis is reflected caudally, the spermatic cords can be identified, each covered in its tunic. A closed castration is performed. The cords are ligated individually just outside the external inguinal rings and then clamped and sectioned distal to the ligatures (see **272–294**). In the photograph, the dog's right spermatic cord has been ligated and sectioned (and is grasped in the nearest hand) and the left cord has been freed from surrounding fascia, prior to ligation.

(**191**) The dorsal penile artery is identified, ligated and clamped. It is then sectioned between the ligature and clamps.

(**192**) The penis is transected just distal to the penile artery ligature and the penis, prepuce, testes and scrotum removed. A urinary catheter is inserted into the urethra.

(**193**) To reduce the risk of postoperative stenosis of the stoma, the urethra is spatulated by incising it ventrally with scissors.

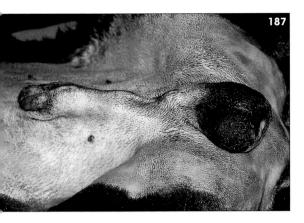

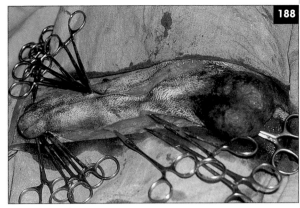

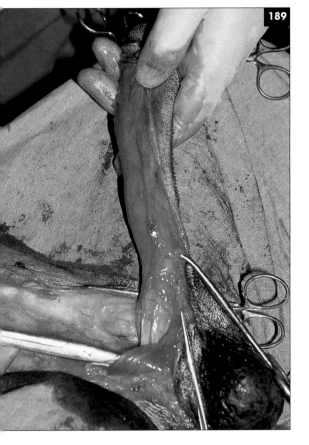

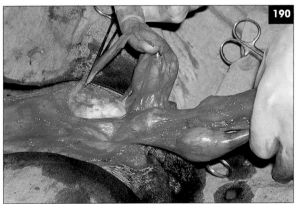

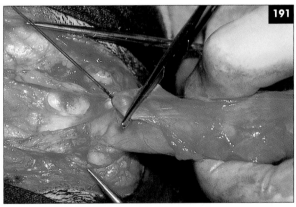

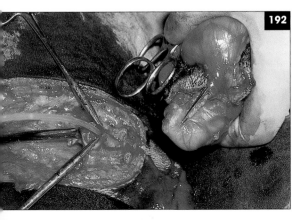

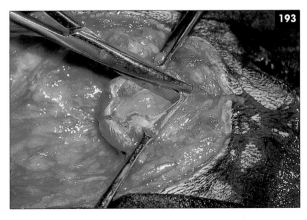

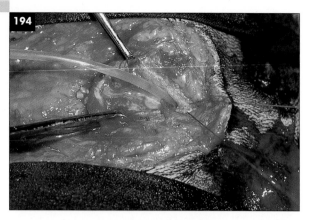

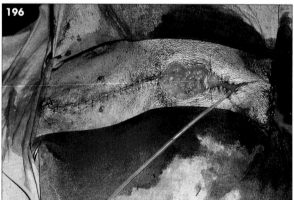

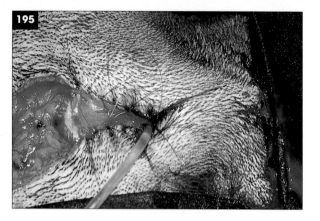

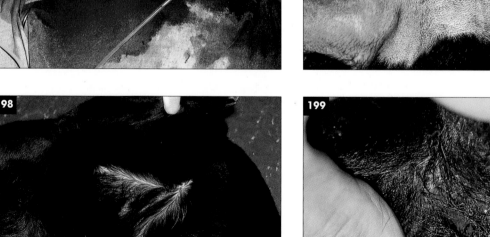

(**194**) A suture of 2/0 synthetic absorbable material is placed between the ventral wall of the urethra at the caudal end of the stoma and the subcutaneous tissues. This is to prevent tension on the suture line after stomatization.

(**195**) The urethral urothelium is sutured to the skin with simple interrupted sutures of 3/0 monofilament nylon.

(**196**) The ventral abdominal subcutaneous tissues and skin cranial to the stoma are closed in separate layers.

(**197**) Closure is completed by suturing the skin to the urethral urothelium at the cranial edge of the stoma.

(**198, 199**) Although it might not be necessary to excise the penis in many cases, the cosmetic effect of this operation is quite good, as can be seen from these follow-up photographs taken three years after surgery. A recent case report described amputation of the penis with preservation of the prepuce (the remaining penile urethral opening is anastomosed to the caudal fornix of the preputial mucosa), but it remains to be proven if this technique provides a more effective barrier to ascending urinary tract infections than conventional urethrostomy techniques.

Bladder displacement usually occurs either ventrally (into an inguinal hernia or ventral rupture) (**200, 201**) or caudally (into a perineal rupture) (**209, 210**). Treatment involves stabilizing the patient, replacement of the organ (**211–213**) and hernia or rupture repair (**202–208** and **214–230**).

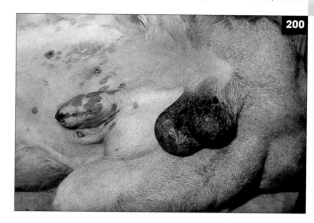

200, 201 This dysuric Old English Sheepdog has bilateral perineal ruptures and a right inguinal hernia (**200**). Retrograde positive contrast urethrocystography revealed that the bladder is displaced into the inguinal hernia (**201**).

202 Diagrammatic representation of inguinal hernia repair. Although twisting of the vaginal tunic during reduction of hernia contents is often recommended (to prevent viscera from re-herniating during reduction and repair), it is not always necessary.

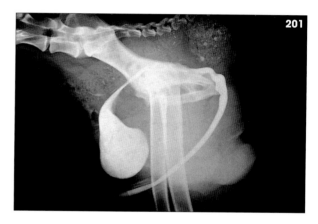

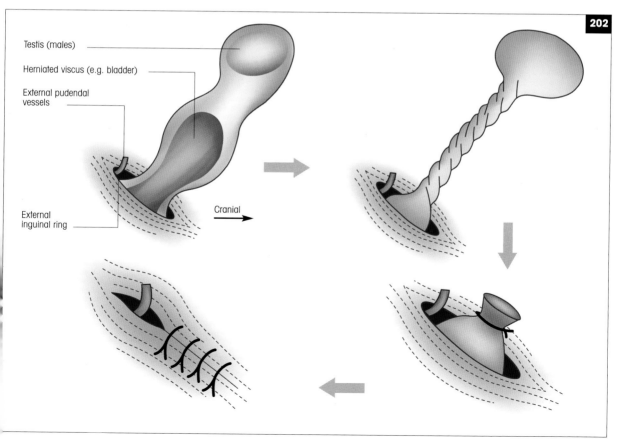

Testis (males)

Herniated viscus (e.g. bladder)

External pudendal vessels

External inguinal ring

Cranial

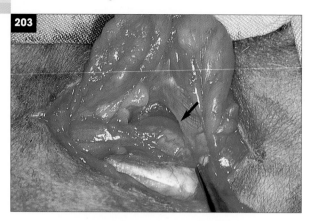

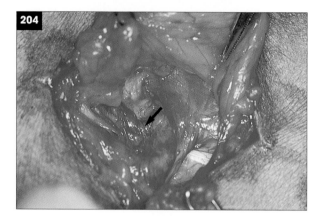

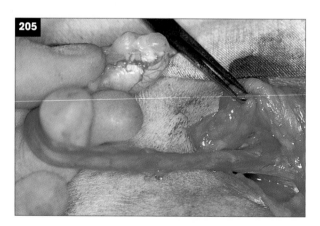

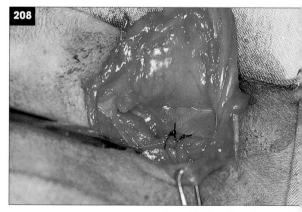

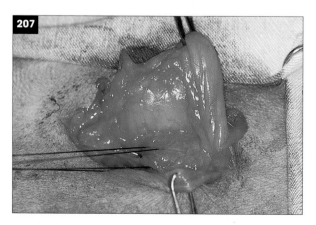

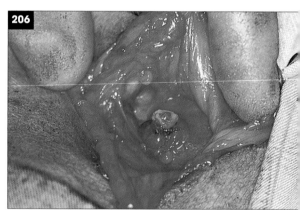

203–208 (**203**) A skin incision is made directly over the hernia and the subcutaneous inguinal fat bluntly separated and reflected medially. In this male Dandie Dinmont, the dog's head is to the right and the penis is below the upper surgical drape. The fat has been reflected medially (upwards in the illustration) to expose the external inguinal ring. The craniomedial part of the ring is formed by the edge of the external abdominal oblique muscle (arrowed). Most of the hernia has been reduced, but some omental fat can still be seen through the vaginal tunic, just to the left of the point of the forceps.

(**204**) When the vaginal tunic is displaced craniolaterally, the large external pudendal vessels can be seen (arrowed). These and their adjacent (invisible) lymphatics must be avoided.

(**205**) The tunic-covered testis and spermatic cord are exteriorized by blunt dissection of fascial attachments and the hernia contents returned to the abdomen (if this has not already been carried out). In the bitch the vaginal tunic sac is freed from surrounding fascial attachments by blunt dissection. In both sexes, care is taken to avoid the external pudendal vessels and their branches, including the caudal epigastric vessels. If the viscera are incarcerated and non-reducible, it may be necessary to incise the proximal vaginal tunic and enlarge the inguinal ring. This is best accomplished by incising the proximal tunic on its cranial border, just distal to the external inguinal ring, and continuing the incision cranially through the external abdominal oblique muscle.

(**206**) After reduction of the hernia contents, a closed castration is performed in male animals (see **272–294**). This effectively obliterates the hernia sac. In bitches, the vaginal tunic is ligated just ventral to the external inguinal ring. The sac is sectioned just distal to the ligature and removed. The ligated sac remnants are now reduced through the inguinal canal.

(**207**) The external inguinal ring is now closed. Simple interrupted sutures of monofilament nylon or synthetic absorbable suture material are used to appose the edges of the external inguinal ring, formed by the caudal edge of the external abdominal oblique muscle craniomedially and the inguinal ligament caudolaterally. Sutures should be pre-placed, as shown, and a 0.5–1.5 cm space left (depending on the size of the animal) at the caudal end of the ring to avoid strangulation of the external pudendal vessels and lymphatics.

(**208**) The sutures are now tied to complete the repair and the gap at the caudal end of the ring checked to ensure that it is large enough to prevent strangulation of vessels and lymphatics but not allow prolapse of viscera adjacent to these structures. The subcutaneous fat, fascia and skin are closed routinely. If a large dead space is present, it is prudent to use a Penrose or active suction drain for 3–5 days to minimize swelling.

209, 210 (**209**) Retroflexion of the urinary bladder into a perineal rupture is not always associated with dysuria. The only sign in this dog was unilateral perineal swelling, which reduced in size during micturition.

(**210**) Retrograde positive contrast urethrocystography (and/or ultrasonography) is the best way of confirming retroflexion of the bladder into a perineal rupture.

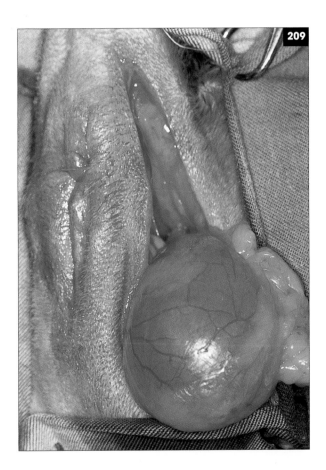

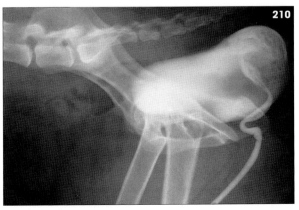

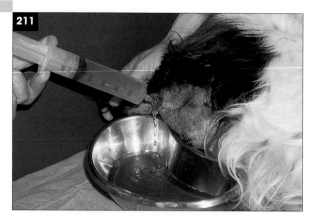

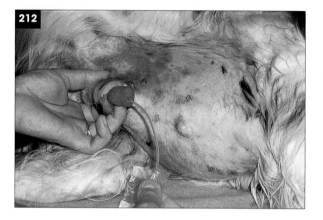

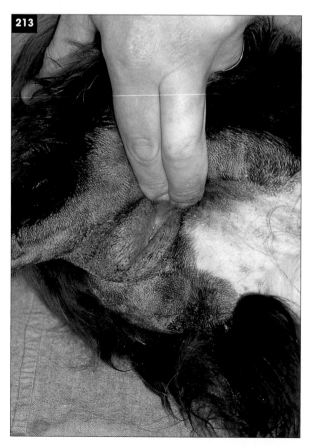

211–213 If retroflexion of the bladder into a perineal rupture results in dysuria, the priority for treatment is relief of the dysuria. It is dangerous to attempt forceful catheterization of the bladder; the tortuous course of the urethra (see **210**) means that iatrogenic trauma by the catheter is highly likely. Initially, therefore, the bladder should be drained by needle centesis through the perineum (**211**). A catheter is then inserted gently *per urethram* to the level of the ischial arch of the urethra (**212**). After drainage by centesis, the bladder can then usually be returned to the abdomen by direct digital pressure through the perineal defect (**213**) and the catheter advanced into it. The catheter is retained as an indwelling catheter for 4–5 days. This allows the bladder and perineum to recover from the effects of bladder entrapment and distension while the animal is treated for the metabolic effects of dysuria. In addition, the use of a polyurethrane catheter, which is soft but stiff, tends to prevent the bladder from returning to the perineum.

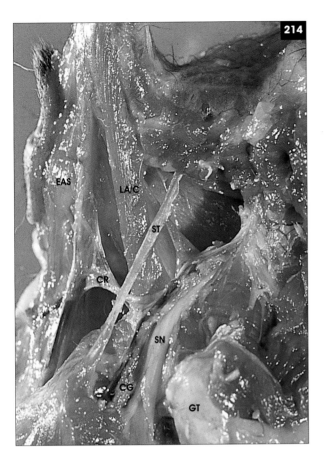

214 For perineal rupture repair, a knowledge of local anatomy is imperative. In this dissection of a dog (positioned as in **215**), the gluteal musculature has been removed from the caudal, right lateral pelvis. The tail has been elevated. Note the position of the following structures and their relationships to each other: EAS = external anal sphincter muscle; LA/C = levator ani (caudomedial)/coccygeus (craniolateral) muscles; CR = caudal rectal (haemorrhoidal) vein, artery and nerve; ST = sacrotuberous ligament; SN = sciatic nerve; CG = caudal gluteal artery and vein; GT = greater trochanter of proximal femur. The breakdown of the perineum usually occurs at the junction between the external anal sphincter and the levator ani muscles (separated on this dissection). Rarely, breakdown occurs between the levator ani and coccygeus muscles.

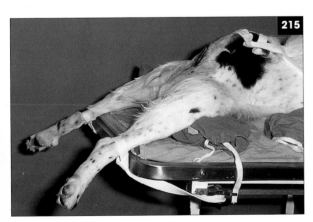

215 The dog should be positioned for surgery in sternal recumbency, with the hind quarters raised by extending the hindlimbs over a sandbag placed under the proximal thighs. The tail should be elevated using tapes.

216, 217 The tails of short-docked breeds are difficult to elevate. In these animals, a large cutting needle can be used to pass no. 2 monofilament nylon ventral to the tail, as illustrated (**216**). The nylon is then tied to itself as a loose loop. Tapes are placed through this loop and used to elevate the remnants of the tail (**217**).

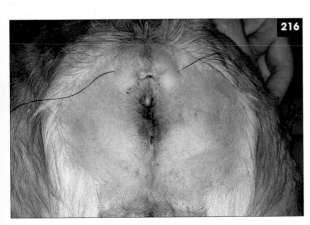

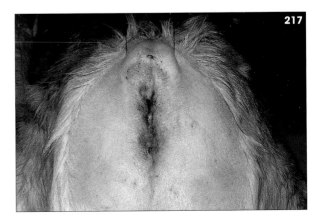

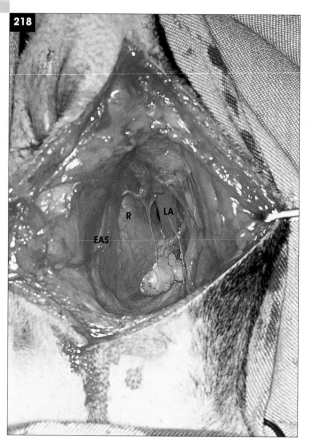

218, 219 The 'best' example of a perineal rupture (**218**). The right perineum has been opened revealing the defect between the external anal sphincter (EAS) and levator ani (LA) muscles into which a rectal deviation (R) protrudes. White, lobulated pelvic fat can be seen on the floor of the pelvis and, beneath this fat, is the internal obturator muscle. It is extremely unusual to be able to see this much anatomy, and so the technique of perineal rupture repair is illustrated below on the type of case more likely to be encountered by the reader. The repair technique is a matter of personal preference (based on experience and results obtained). It is well-recognized that different surgeons, apparently performing an identical repair technique, get different results and so, if one finds a method which works, one tends to stick with it. While the use of an internal obturator muscle flap is popular for the repair, the author prefers the technique of re-apposing the external anal sphincter to the levator ani cranially (but including the sacrotuberous ligament in the sutures) and to the internal obturator muscle ventrally. This is summarized in the diagram (**219**), although only three sutures are shown in this figure.

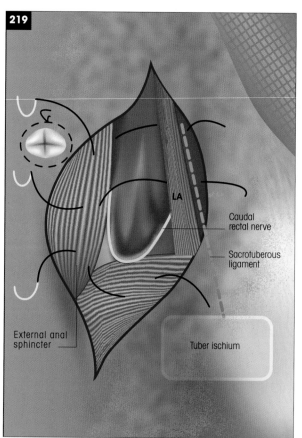

Caudal
rectal nerve

Sacrotuberous
ligament

LA

External anal
sphincter

Tuber ischium

220–230 (**220**) This is a more typical case. The animal has been anaesthetized, its rectum evacuated of faeces and the anal sacs emptied. The dog is positioned for surgery in ventral recumbency with the hindlimbs extended caudally over a sandbag and the tail elevated (see **215**). A temporary purse-string suture is used to close the anus. After routine aseptic skin preparation and draping, an incision is made just lateral to the region of the external anal sphincter muscle. This can frequently be judged by palpating the defect in the perineum but, if not, the skin is incised just lateral to the lateral margin of the glandular circumanal skin, which corresponds to the lateral edges of the external anal sphincter muscle. The incision is extended ventrally to a level just above the pelvic floor (this can be judged by palpating the tuber ischium on the affected side). The subcutaneous fat and fascia are separated by blunt dissection and the perineal defect exposed. This dog has a right-sided perineal rupture with no anatomy visible apart from fat and fascia. This is fairly typical.

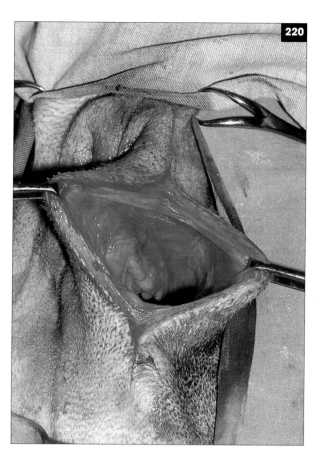

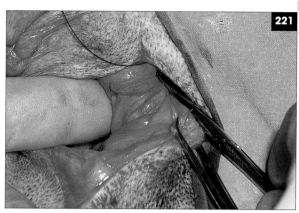

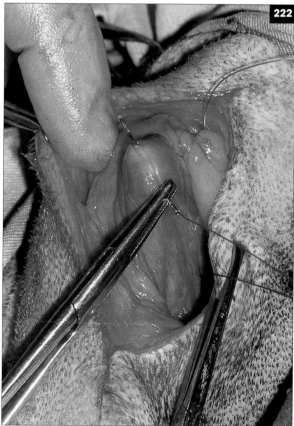

(**221**) Here, an index finger has been inserted into the defect, medial to the levator ani muscle. The sacro-tuberous ligament is palpated through the muscle; this is always possible, even when the muscle is not visible, as in this case. With the ball of the finger on the ligament, the finger tip is bent slightly ventrally and laterally into a small depression. A pulse should now be palpable by the tip of the finger. This pulse is in the caudal gluteal artery and gives an indication of how close the sciatic nerve and caudal gluteal vessels are to the ligament (refer to **214**). A curved round-bodied suture needle with swaged-on No. 0 monofilament polyamide is inserted dorsally, lateral to the ligament. Taking care to stay as close to the ligament as possible, the needle is curved cranially around the ligament. Automatically, the tip of the needle exits medially through the levator ani muscle remnants. The needle tip is palpated as it emerges from the levator ani muscle and is braced against the finger tip. This is to prevent the needle point from damaging the rectum and also to avoid losing it in the lateral pelvic soft tissues when the needle holders are released. The needle holders are now used to grip close to the point of the needle and pull the suture around the sacrotuberous ligament.

(**222**) The external anal sphincter muscle is now identified beneath the medial part of the skin incision. The muscle is usually visible but, if not, its position can be determined by placing an index finger on the lateral wall of the rectum and curling it caudally until a thickening is appreciated. This is the cranial edge of the external anal sphincter muscle. A bite is now taken through the cranial edge of the muscle, as shown.

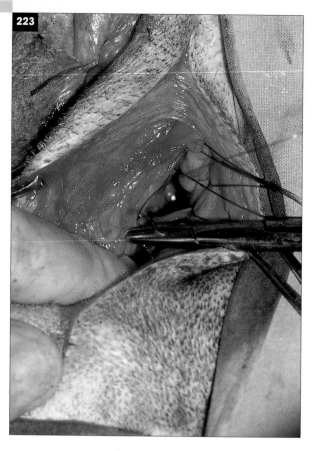

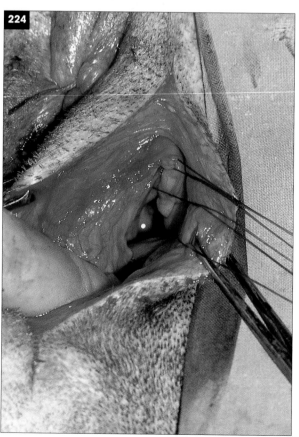

(**223**) Sutures continue to be pre-placed between the sacrotuberous ligament and the external anal sphincter muscle, as described above. However, care should be taken to avoid placing sutures around or through the caudal rectal nerve as it enters the external anal sphincter muscle. The location of this nerve can usually be identified by detecting the pulse in its adjacent artery but, if not, it should be assumed to be entering the sphincter at the '8 o'clock' (left side) or '4 o'clock' (right side) positions on the cranial edge of the sphincter muscle. The nerve is not apparent in this dog, but the needle holders are being used to point to the location of its entry into the sphincter. This area must be avoided during suture placement, as illustrated by the position of the middle of the three sutures in **219**.

(**224**) When the last suture has been placed between the ventral end of the sacrotuberous ligament (close to its insertion into the tuber ischium) and the external anal sphincter muscle, a defect remains in the ventral perineum, as shown. This can be closed by suturing the external anal sphincter muscle to the internal obturator muscle.

(**225**) A suture is placed in the internal obturator muscle, as shown. The suture enters the muscle caudal to the internal pudendal vessels (the pulse in the artery can be palpated on the pelvic floor overlying the internal obturator muscle). It is preferable to insert the needle in a craniocaudal direction, as illustrated. This is slightly more difficult than passing the needle lateromedially, but greatly reduces the risk of trauma to the urethra. If the muscle cannot be seen, the needle is passed ventrally until it contacts the bone of the ischium and is then continued caudally and dorsally to exit the muscle. In doing so, it has to have passed in and out of the internal obturator muscle.

(**226**) If one is unsure of the suture placement in the internal obturator muscle, tension should be applied to the suture, as illustrated. If the suture has passed through fat and fascia only, it will tear out and should be replaced.

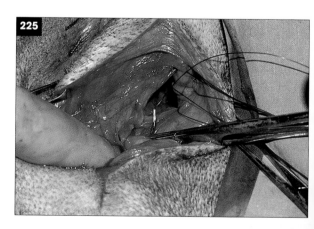

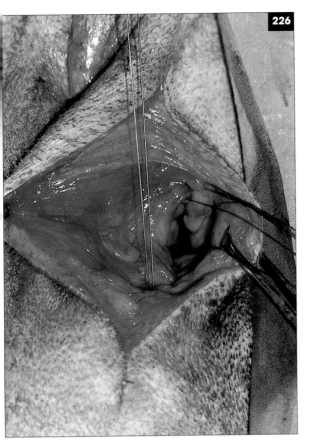

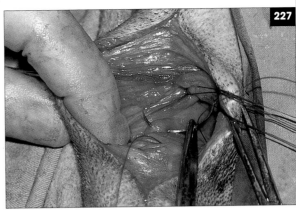

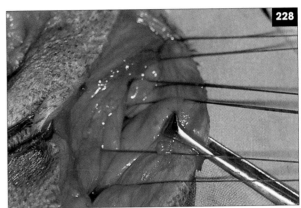

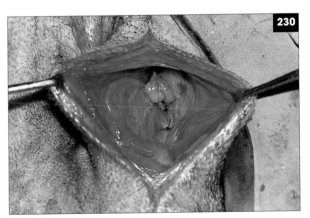

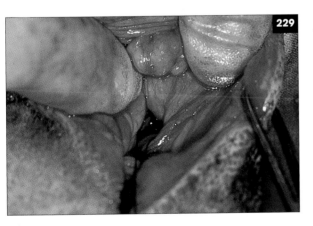

(**227**) The suture is then taken through the ventral part of the cranial edge of the external anal sphincter muscle, taking care to avoid the caudal rectal nerve.
(**228**) When all the sutures have been placed, they can be tied. The author prefers to commence at the ventral part of the defect, since this tends to prevent viscera such as pelvic fat from prolapsing through the defect as the remaining sutures are tied.
(**229**) Care should be taken to tie all sutures tight. The dorsal-most sutures in a large dog will be tied some 6–8 cm from the perineal skin wound edges and so finger tip tightening of the suture knots at this depth is required, as shown.

(**230**) Once the muscular defect has been closed (illustrated), the remaining tissues are apposed. The fascia is closed with a simple continuous synthetic absorbable suture. Frequently, there is little fat and fascia medially. In this case, the lateral fat and fascia are sutured to the superficial fibres of the external anal sphincter muscle. The skin is closed routinely and the purse-string suture removed from the anus. The dog can now be repositioned and castrated (see **272–294**).

Occasionally, animals are presented in which the dysuria appears to be a functional disorder. This is usually associated with an inability of the bladder to contract (bladder atony) or/and a failure of the urethra to relax during attempts to micturate (dyssynergia). Bladder atony may result from a previous bout of dysuria and urinary retention causing overdistension of the bladder. The bladder may appear large and atonic (like a partly inflated football) during contrast radiography. Such overdistension, especially if acute, results in bladder wall ischaemia (see **2** and **135**), breakdown of tight junctions and stretching (and thus demyelination) of nerves coursing over the bladder wall. All of these may result in a loss of function. If severe, this may be irreversible. Such cases are best treated by keeping the bladder empty for 5–10 days, using an indwelling urethral catheter (see **89–91**). This may allow tight junctions to reform and remyelination of nerves to occur, and improves blood flow within the bladder wall. In the author's experience, cholinergic drugs such as bethanechol are rarely effective in these cases. Dyssynergia can be voluntary (a failure of urethral striated muscle to relax) or involuntary (a failure of relaxation of urethral smooth muscle) and is difficult to diagnose. In theory, urodynamics should be beneficial for confirming the diagnosis but, in the absence of patient cooperation and the need for sedation/anaesthesia, it is difficult to interpret the results. The diagnosis usually rests on the history and elimination of physical or neurological causes for the dysuria by imaging and laboratory examinations. Voluntary dyssynergia may be seen in bitches after colposuspension; it responds rapidly to diazepam (0.2 mg/kg p/o bid or tid, given 20–30 minutes before exercising the dog to urinate). Idiopathic dyssynergia is commoner in large breed male dogs such as Labrador Retrievers and may be difficult to treat. If there is no response to treatment for voluntary dyssynergia using diazepam or other striated muscle relaxants, therapy for involuntary dyssynergia using α-adrenergic blocking agents such as phenoxybenzamine hydrochloride (for dogs, 0.25 mg/kg p/o bid or tid) can be attempted. The response may be poor and some affected dogs require long-term management using tube cystostomies (**231–234**).

In a few of these dogs, normal function may return and so, periodically, the owners should leave the cystostomy tube capped for 8–12 hours and observe if the animal is able to urinate and how much urine is passed. The success of apparent urination should be checked by draining what urine is left in the bladder after urination (via the tube) and reporting the residual volume to the veterinary surgeon, who can then assess the efficacy of urination.

Rarely, enlargement of other, adjacent viscera may cause pressure on the urethra or bladder neck, leading to dysuria. Examples are ureterocoeles (**235, 236**), vaginal floor tumours (**237, 238**) or cysts (**239–244**) and sublumbar lymph node enlargement (**245**). Even rarer is congenital narrowing of the genital tract impairing urine outflow (**246, 247**).

231 Tube cystostomy in a male dog using a Foley catheter (photograph taken at the time of tube removal).

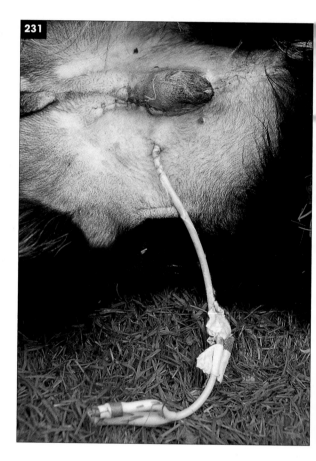

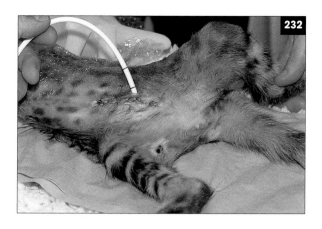

232–234 (**232**) Mushroom tip catheters are preferred to Foley catheters for tube cystostomies. They have the advantage that they can be shortened after insertion and are less likely to come out prematurely. If they are difficult to remove, the mushroom tip (**233**) can be distorted into a more linear shape by carefully inserting a blunt probe and stretching the tip (**234**) during removal.

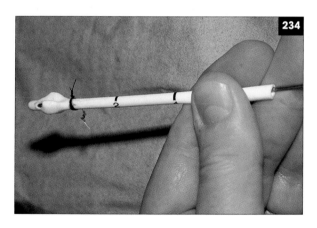

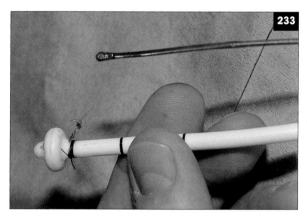

235, 236 Ectopic ureterocoele demonstrated during IVU (**235**). If these become large enough, they can obstruct the bladder neck (**236**).

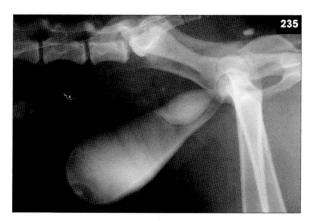

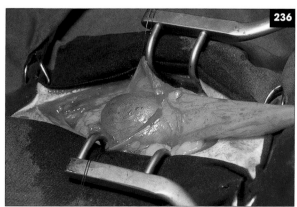

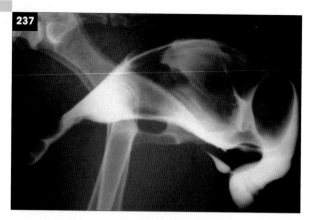

237

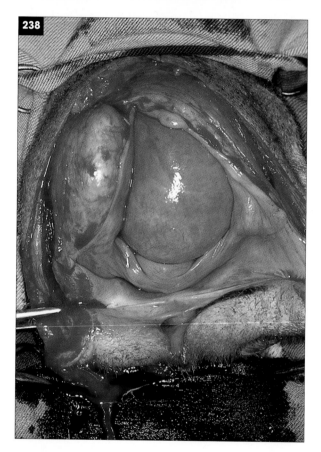

238

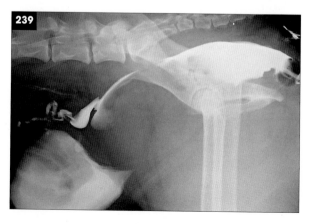

239

237, 238 Extensive vaginal neoplasms demonstrated by retrograde vaginography (**237**) and during episiotomy (**238**) in a Cocker Spaniel bitch. Depending on their size and position, these may compress the distal urethra or inhibit exit of urine from the vagina (**238**), but this is rare. These tumours are usually leiomyomas or, rarely, leiomyosarcomas or carcinomas.

239 Vagino-urethrogram (performed shortly after IVU) of an adult Airedale bitch presented with dysuria. A soft-tissue density can be seen in the ventral part of the vaginal lumen, extending cranially and compressing the urethra and bladder neck. Ultrasonography revealed that this was a fluid-filled swelling. Bacteriological and cytological examinations of the fluid confirmed that this was a vaginal wall cyst.

240–244 Vaginal floor cysts can be marsupialized into the vagina via an episiotomy. The bitch is placed in ventral recumbency with the hindquarters raised over a sandbag, as in perineal rupture repair (see **215**). The tail is elevated and the perineum prepared for aseptic surgery.
(**240**) The anus is closed using a purse-string suture. A vertical skin incision is made, extending from just ventral to the external anal sphincter muscle to the dorsal commissure of the vulval lips.
(**241**) The incision is continued through the dorsal vaginal wall using scissors.
(**242**) The urethra is catheterized. The cyst can be seen bulging into the vagina just cranial to the external urethral orifice.
(**243**) The vaginal mucosa over the cyst is incised, revealing the cyst wall, as shown. The cyst wall is then incised and the cyst drained.

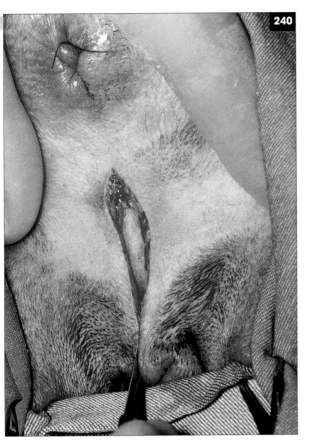

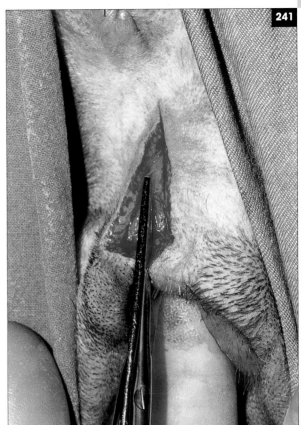

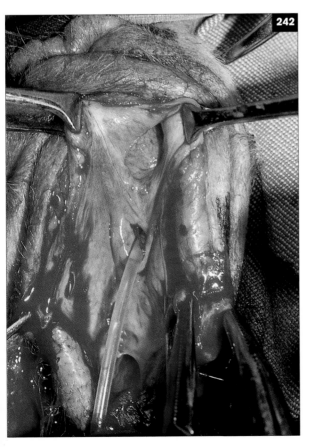

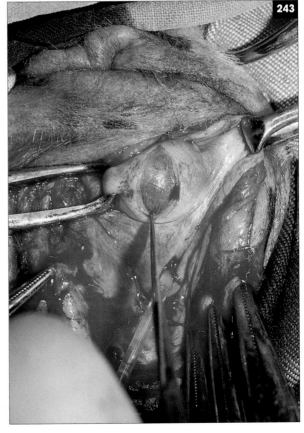

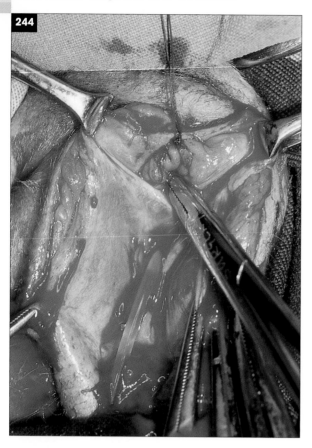

(**244**) The cyst and vaginal mucosal incisions are then apposed using a simple continuous pattern of synthetic absorbable suture material, resulting in a stoma between the cyst and vaginal lumina (the tip of the Kilner needle holder has been inserted into the stoma). Repair of the episiotomy is routine and involves closure of the dorsal vaginal wall using synthetic absorbable material in a simple continuous pattern, followed by simple interrupted sutures of monofilament nylon in the skin. The purse-string suture is then removed from the anus. The urethral catheter is also removed unless there is the possibility of postoperative dysuria resulting from urethral or peri-urethral swelling, in which case it can be sutured *in situ* as an indwelling catheter (see **89, 90**).

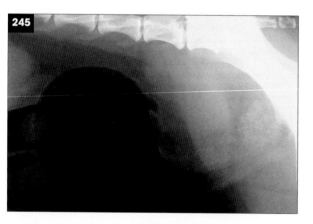

245 Sublumbar lymph node enlargement (lymphosarcoma) resulting in bladder neck and rectal compression, demonstrated radiographically (a pneumocystogram has been performed to demonstrate the position of the bladder). This dog exhibited dysuria and dyschezia.

246, 247 Congenital narrowing of the preputial orifice in a puppy resulting in dysuria (**246**). During urination, the prepuce filled with urine, which then gradually dripped out through the tiny preputial orifice. This was treated by spatulation (**247**) to give the dog a larger orifice.

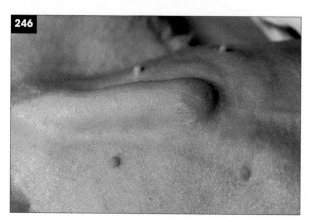

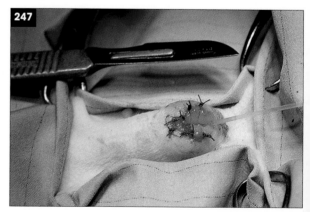

5 Prostatic disorders

Within the hallowed gland...
Dylan Thomas (1914–1953)

Diagnosis

PROSTATE DISORDERS in small animals are most common in the dog. Prostate disorders in cats are extremely uncommon, although cats will occasionally develop prostatic malignancies. Problems affecting the canine prostate include:

- Benign enlargement (hyperplasia/metaplasia).
- Prostatitis (acute or chronic).
- Abscessation.
- Prostatic cysts – intraprostatic (prostatic retention cysts) or paraprostatic.
- Neoplasia (usually adenocarcinoma, although it may be difficult to differentiate primary prostate cancer from urethral carcinomas invading the prostate gland without histopathology).
- Idiopathic haemorrhage.
- Displacement of the prostate into ruptures or hernias.
- Trauma.

The clinical signs in dogs with prostate disorders include haematuria, dysuria, urinary incontinence, dyschezia, pain and weight loss. These signs are not pathognomonic and so must be differentiated from similar signs due to non-prostatic disorders. A useful sign is if the dog bleeds from the urethra between micturitions (see **5**). This suggests that the haemorrhage is coming from distal to the bladder neck, most commonly from the prostate, although the urethra, penis and prepuce should be examined to eliminate other areas of possible haemorrhage. Once it is known that the signs are associated with a prostatic condition, the nature of that condition should be determined.

Palpation of the prostate is best performed using two hands (see **9**). Useful differential features are that only acute prostatitis (± abscessation) and neoplasia are painful conditions; prostatic abscesses, cysts and tumours result in asymmetrical prostatic enlargement (*Table 11*); in some dogs with prostatic tumours a small, irregular, painful prostate is present.

Table 11 **Differential clinical findings in prostate disorders**

	Enlarged	Symmetrical	Painful	Firm (FM) or Fluctuating (FL)	Urethral discharge (nature of any discharge)
Hyperplasia/metaplasia	+	+	−	FM	± (semen)
Prostatitis	±	+	+	FM	± (blood, pus)
Abscessation	+	−	+	FL	± (pus)
Cysts	+	−	−	FL	−
Neoplasia	±	±	+	FM	−
Idiopathic haemorrhage	−	+	−	FM	+ (blood)

+   usually present
−   usually absent
±   may be present or absent

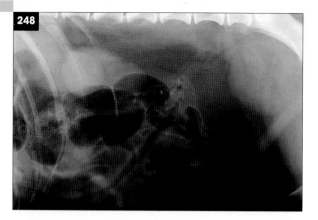

Prostate cancer is also one of the few (if not the only) prostate conditions to affect castrated dogs. Indeed, some authors believe prostate cancer to have a higher prevalence in castrated versus entire animals. As with any suspected malignancy, examination for metastases is mandatory (see 20). Animals with prostate cancer (and other intrapelvic malignancies) will sometimes have abnormal periosteal reactions on the bones of the pelvis, femurs and/or the ventral lumbar and lumbosacral vertebrae (see 21, 22).

Apart from clinical examination, useful investigative techniques include contrast radiography (especially retrograde positive contrast urethrocystography), ultrasonography, fine needle aspirates and biopsies, cytology and histology (see 69 and 248–263).

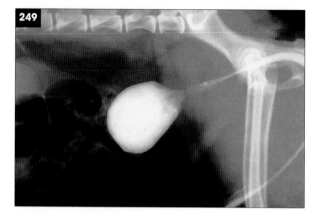

248, 249 The enlarged prostate visible on the plain lateral abdominal radiograph (248) of this Springer Spaniel shows asymmetry during retrograde positive contrast urethrography (249), with more prostatic tissue dorsal to the urethra than ventral to it. This was due to an intraprostatic abscess.

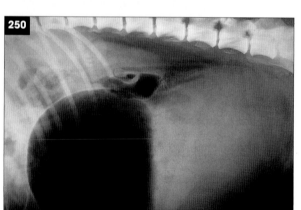

250, 251 The gas-filled bladder in this dog (250) is due to gas-producing organisms. The dog had retention cystitis associated with the enlarged prostate gland. The gland shows asymmetry during urethrography (251). This dog had a large intraprostatic cyst.

252 Urethrocystogram of the dog illustrated in 20–22. The gross spillage of contrast medium into irregular cavities within the prostate is almost pathognomonic for prostatic or prostatic urethral malignancy.

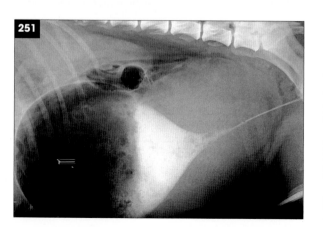

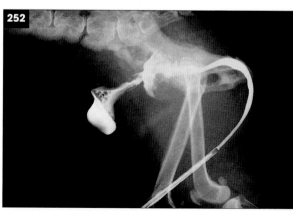

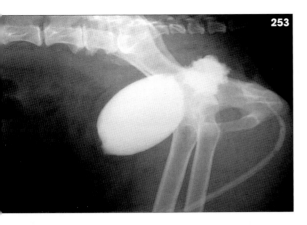

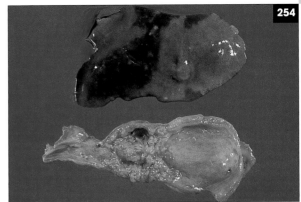

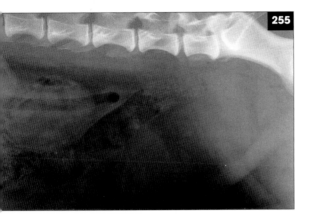

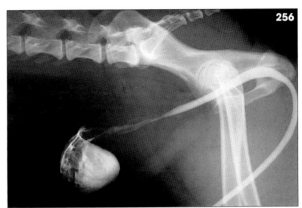

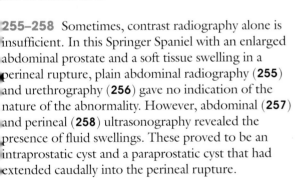

253, 254 A further example of prostatic cavitation in a dog associated with malignancy (**253**). The postmortem appearance and the pulmonary metastases can be seen in **254**.

255–258 Sometimes, contrast radiography alone is insufficient. In this Springer Spaniel with an enlarged abdominal prostate and a soft tissue swelling in a perineal rupture, plain abdominal radiography (**255**) and urethrography (**256**) gave no indication of the nature of the abnormality. However, abdominal (**257**) and perineal (**258**) ultrasonography revealed the presence of fluid swellings. These proved to be an intraprostatic cyst and a paraprostatic cyst that had extended caudally into the perineal rupture.

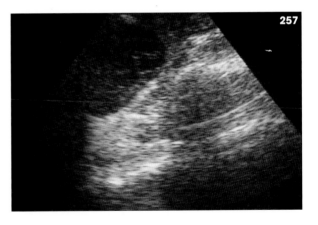

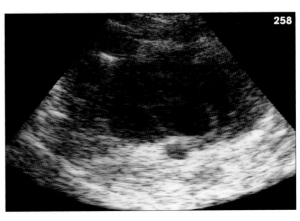

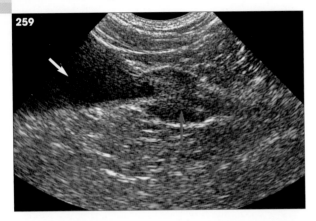

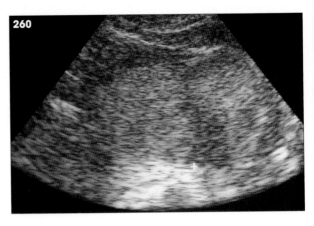

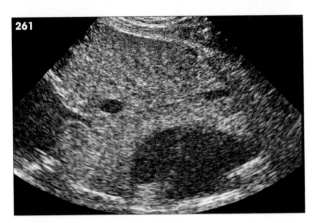

259 The ultrasonographic appearance of a normal canine prostate (red arrow) in longitudinal section. (The urinary bladder is indicated by a white arrow.) Note that the prostate tissue is homogeneous.

260 The ultrasonographic appearance of a normal canine prostate in transverse section. The gland tissue is homogeneous and the lobes are symmetrical in size and shape.

261 Ultrasonographic appearance of canine intraprostatic cysts (centesis and fluid cytology/bacteriology would be needed to differentiate these definitively from abscesses).

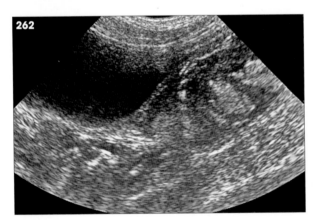

262 Ultrasonographic appearance of a canine prostatic malignancy, showing heterogenicity and asymmetry.

263 Ultrasonography makes aspiration of the contents of prostatic cysts and abscesses more accurate and safer.

Treatment

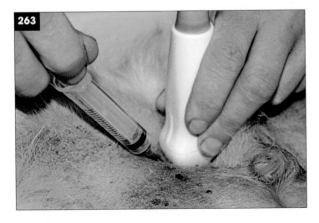

IF THE PROSTATE DISORDER results in dysuria, the priority is to alleviate the dysuria before diagnosis and treatment of the disorder (see Chapter 4 and **264**).

Benign prostatic enlargement is usually due to acinar hyperplasia associated with an excess of androgens, although oestrogens can also lead to prostatic enlargement, since they result in squamous metaplasia (particularly of the ducts) and fibromuscular hyperplasia of the gland stroma. If severe, the squamous metaplasia of the ducts may result in duct obstruction and retention of prostatic secretions, leading to retention (intraprostatic) cysts. Prostatic hyperplasia responds to oestrogen or anti-androgen therapy (**265–271**) and, more permanently, to castration (**272–294**).

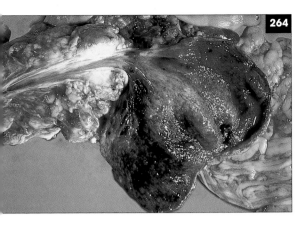

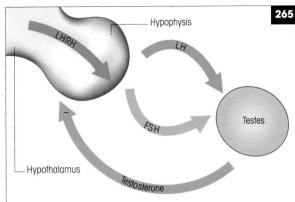

264 Postmortem appearance of prostate cancer in a dog. This resulted in obstructive dysuria leading to bladder ischaemia, the effects of which can be seen. The priority in this case would have been to relieve the pressure within the bladder (see Chapter 4).

265 In the normal animal, luteinizing hormone releasing hormone (LHRH) from the hypothalamus stimulates release of the gonadotrophins luteinizing hormone (LH) and follicle stimulating hormone (FSH) from the hypophysis. LH has the effect on the testes of stimulating testosterone production. There is a negative feedback mechanism on the hypophysis, so that increasing levels of testosterone reduce the amount of LHRH, thus keeping testosterone levels in check.

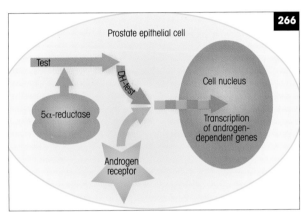

266 In the prostate epithelial cells, testosterone (Test) is converted into dihydrotestosterone (DHtest) by the enzyme 5α-reductase. DHtest is about twice as potent as Test; it has greater binding affinity for and slower dissociation from intracellular androgen receptors. Within the nucleus, the DHtest–androgen receptor complex interacts with specific DNA binding sites and initiates transcription of androgen-dependent genes. The resultant messenger RNA is translated and cellular protein increased. In the prostate this leads to cellular hypertrophy and hyperplasia of the epithelial component of the gland.

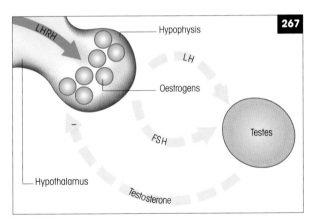

267, 268 The action of oestrogens. Oestrogens are sometimes used to treat prostatic hyperplasia. Their action is to suppress LHRH release, block androgen receptors and inhibit 5α-reductase. Long-term oestrogen therapy should be used with caution. Apart from potential toxicity effects, it may lead to prostatic enlargement due to squamous metaplasia and fibromuscular hypoplasia.

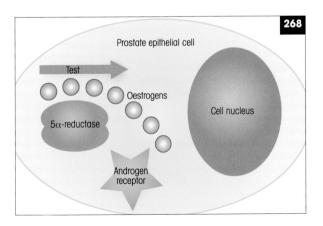

269, 270 Steroidal anti-androgens such as delmadinone acetate are used for the medical treatment of prostatic hyperplasia. Their action is to suppress release of LHRH and block androgen receptors.

271 In breeding males, it may be tempting to use 5α-reductase inhibitors such as finasteride to preserve circulating testosterone levels (and thus libido). However, there is a possibility that these drugs may be teratogenic.

272–287 Castration with retention of the scrotum. (**272**) The anaesthetized dog is positioned in dorsal recumbency, with the hindlimbs abducted. The scrotum and surrounding skin are prepared for aseptic surgery, avoiding the use of strong antiseptics such as surgical spirit if the scrotum is to be retained. The area is draped (caudal is to the left in this photograph). (**273**) To avoid postoperative scrotal skin irritation, the skin incision is made prescrotally. The second finger of the left hand (if one is right-handed) is used to push one of the testes to a prescrotal position. (**274**) While the second finger maintains the testis in that position, the first finger and thumb are used to tense the testis upwards and immobilize it against the prescotal skin. (**275**) The skin and subcutaneous fascia are incised to expose the tunica vaginalis over the testis. Usually, a small amount of fat (external to the tunic) appears in the incision site when the incision has reached the required depth. The fat can be seen at the cranial end of the incision. (**276**) The thumb and index finger of both hands are used to apply pressure beneath and thus exteriorize the testis. (**277**) The testis is grasped firmly in the left hand and the cremaster muscle and tunic-covered vas deferens and pampiniform plexus are identified at the cranial end of the testis. (**278**) A dry swab is used to push fascia proximally from the lateral side of the testis. (**279**) The same procedure is used to debride the medial side of the testis.

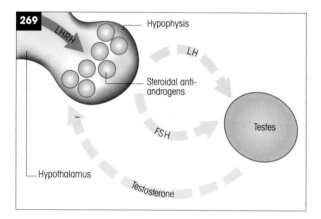

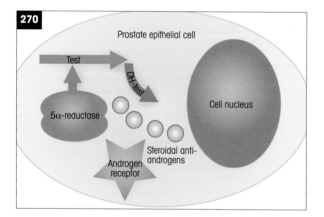

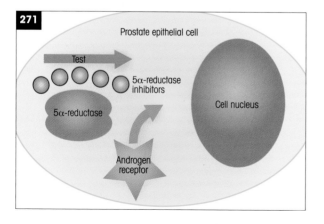

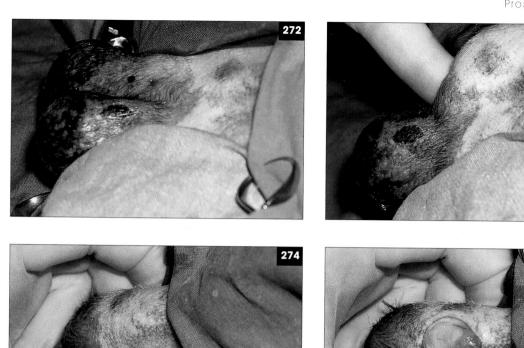

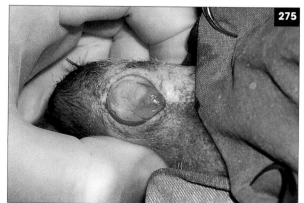

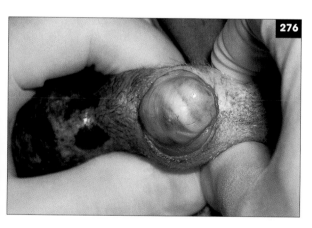

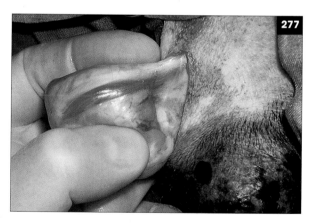

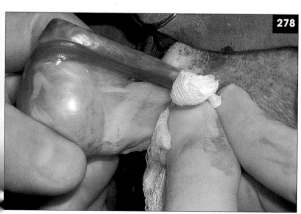

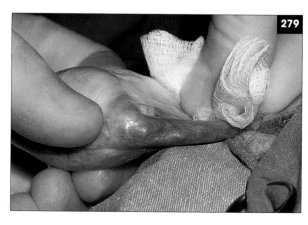

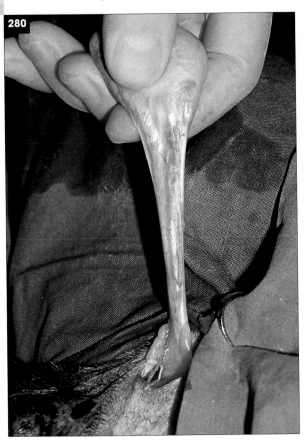

(**280**) The gubernaculum can now easily be broken down and the testis and spermatic cord exteriorized, as shown.

(**281**) Any remaining fascia is cleared from the tunic over the spermatic cord by wiping with a swab from distally to proximally.

(**282**) The spermatic cord is now ligated. The author prefers to use a transfixing ligature of synthetic absorbable material. It is important that transfixing ligatures do not enter hollow viscera (such as, in this case, the vas deferens) in order to avoid the risk of granuloma formation. The ligature is therefore taken through the tunic and between the spermatic vessels (cranially) and the vas (caudally), as illustrated.

(**283**) The ligature is tied cranially to ligate the spermatic vessels.

(**284**) The ends of the ligature are then taken caudally, around each side of the spermatic cord, and again tied.

(**285**) The result is that during placement of the transfixing ligature the vascular component of the spermatic cord is ligated twice, thus minimizing the risk of haemorrhage.

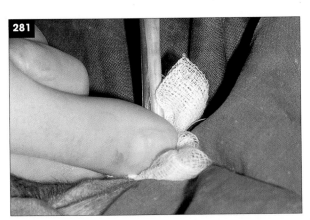

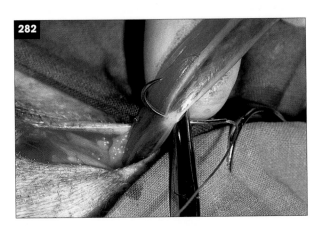

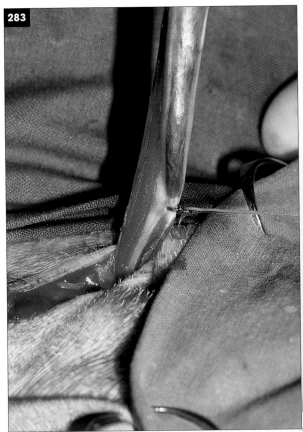

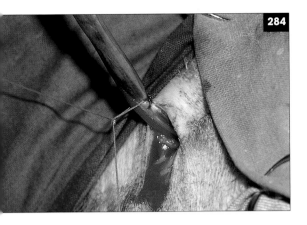

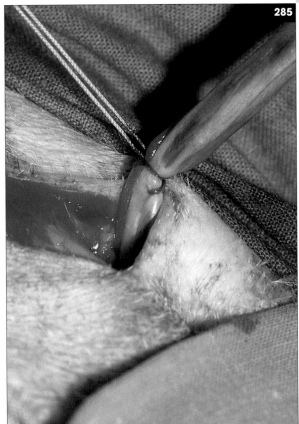

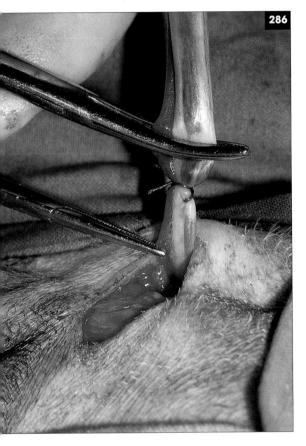

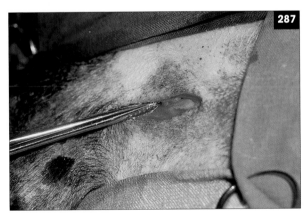

(286) Vascular clamps are applied to the spermatic cord just distal to the ligature. A second pair of clamps is used to grasp a caudal, non-vascular part of the spermatic cord (in this case the cremaster muscle). The spermatic cord is sectioned between the ligature and the first pair of clamps and the testis is removed.

(287) The ligated spermatic cord is allowed to retract through the incision towards the external inguinal ring. The adequacy of the ligation is unknown until this stage since, even if the ligature has not been placed tight enough, the tension on the spermatic vessels while the testis is exteriorized may prevent haemorrhage from occuring. If haemorrhage does occur when the tension on the spermatic cord remnants is released, the cord can be re-exteriorized using the forceps and religated. If, as should happen, no haemorrhage occurs, the forceps are removed. Castration is completed by displacing the remaining testis cranially to the skin incision, incising the common vaginal tunic and repeating the procedure described above. The skin and subcutaneous fascia are then closed routinely.

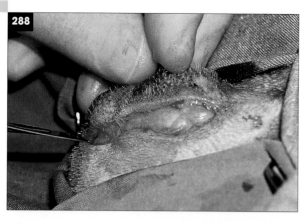

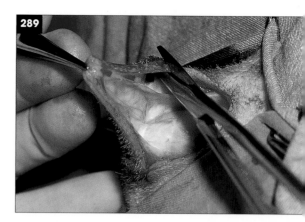

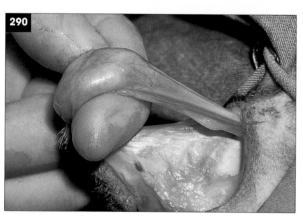

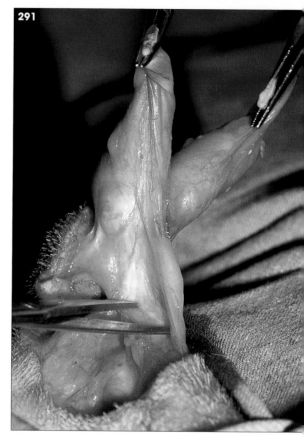

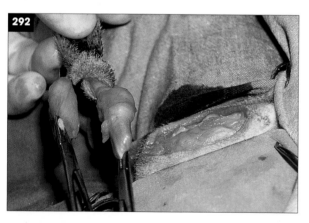

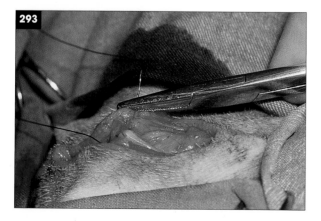

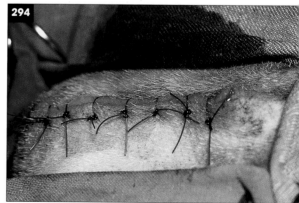

288–294 Castration including scrotal ablation.
(**288**) The dog is positioned and the surgical site prepared as in **272**. An eliptical skin incision is made around the base of the scrotum.
(**289**) The subcuticular fascia is undermined and incised, freeing the edges of the scrotal skin. Any bleeding subcutaneous tissue vessels are ligated or cauterized using diathermy.
(**290**) Each testis is identified within its tunic. Its spermatic cord is cleared of extraneous fascia, ligated and sectioned, as described in **286**.
(**291**) After both cords have been ligated, the remaining fascia is separated by blunt and sharp dissection.
(**292**) The testes and scrotum can now be removed.
(**293**) The subcutaneous fascia is closed using a simple continuous suture pattern of synthetic absorbable material.
(**294**) The skin wound is closed routinely, in this case with simple interrupted monofilament polypropylene sutures. A subcuticular suture of synthetic absorbable material would also be suitable.

The vast majority of prostatic tumours are malignant (usually adenocarcinomas), with local and distant invasion and spread (see **20–22**, **252–254** and **295–299**) and the prognosis is hopeless.

295 Extensive local spread of a prostatic tumour in a dog. Note the appearance of the bladder due to ischaemia after the urethral obstruction and bladder distension caused by the tumour.

296–299 Prostatic adenocarcinoma in a cat demonstrated by lateral (**296**) and ventrodorsal (**297**) radiographs during urethrography. The postmortem appearance is shown in **298** and **299**. Note the cavitation of the prostate gland and the local extension of the tumour into surrounding tissues, and also the similarities to the canine condition (see **252–254**).

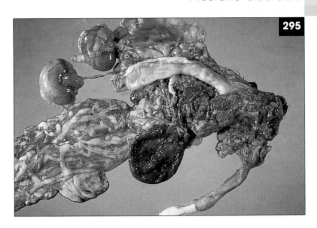

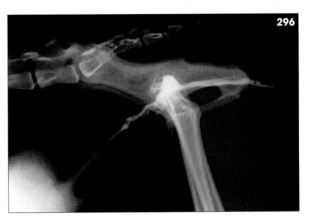

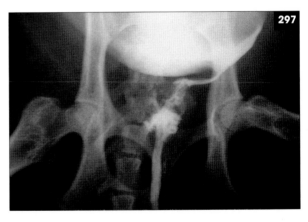

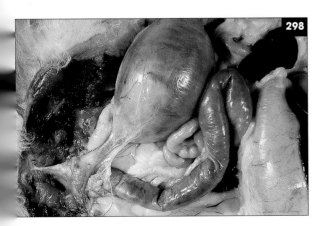

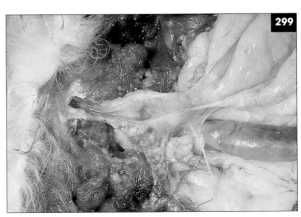

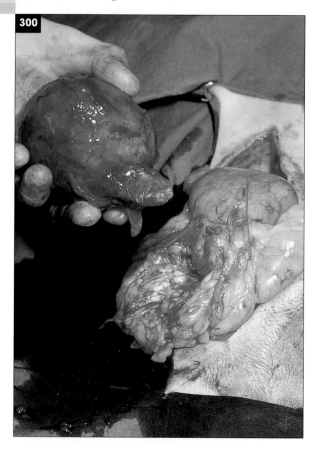

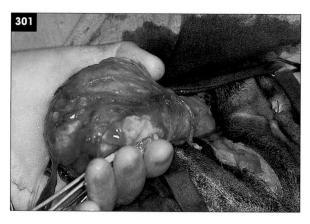

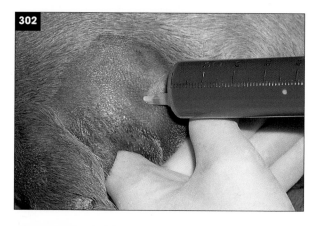

Prostatectomy in dogs with prostatic malignancy is not to be recommended in the author's view, although some palliation may be obtained in some animals with NSAIDs, particularly cyclo-oxygenase inhibitors such as piroxicam or meloxicam. Other palliative measures (mainly in dysuric dogs) include the use of transurethral resection, partial prostatectomy (either surgical or using a Nd:YAG laser) tube cystostomies (see **231–234**) and/or urethral stents. Unlike the situation in humans, oestrogen or anti-androgen therapy or castration appear to have no beneficial effects in increasing the quality of life or longevity in dogs with prostate cancer.

Mild prostatitis may respond to antibiotics and castration, but abscesses and cysts require surgical drainage. The prognosis associated with prostatic cysts and abscesses is guarded and no one form of treatment is 100% successful. Treatment of prostatic cysts and abscesses has included excision (**300**, **301**), repeated needle drainage and castration (**302**), Penrose drainage, marsupialization (**303–308**), tube drainage (**309–312**) and omentalization ± partial resection (**313–317**).

300, 301 Pedunculated, canine paraprostatic cysts being excised from the abdomen (**300**) and a perineal rupture (**301**). Great care needs to be taken during excision of intra-abdominal cysts in order to avoid damage to the ureters (which may be adherent to the cyst) and the blood and nerve supplies to the bladder and urethra.

302 Needle drainage of a prostatic abscess in a perineal rupture. In cases of small, intraprostatic cysts or abscesses, repeated needle drainage and castration may resolve the problem.

303–305 (**303**) During marsupialization, the cyst/abscess is stomatized to the skin adjacent to the prepuce. Note the appearance of the tissue of the cyst wall in this dog; this proved to be a carcinoma of the cyst lining and the dog was euthanased three weeks later.
(**304**) In most cases (as in this dog), the cyst/abscess cavity is obliterated and the stoma heals. However, in some dogs the stoma remains patent, draining a tacky, serous secretion for the remainder of the dog's life.
(**305**) Prostatic cysts/abscesses in the perineum, which cannot be excised or returned to the abdomen for omentalization, can be marsupialized into the perineum.

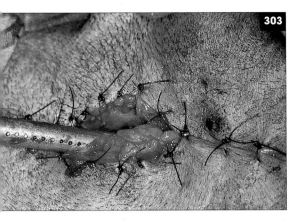

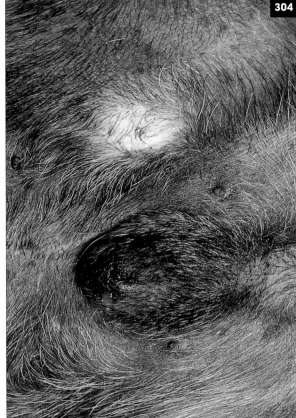

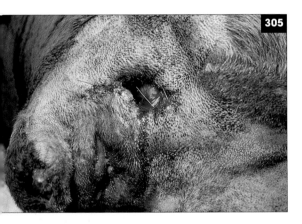

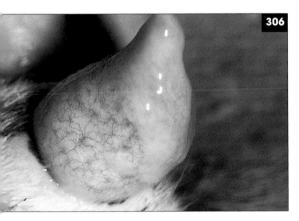

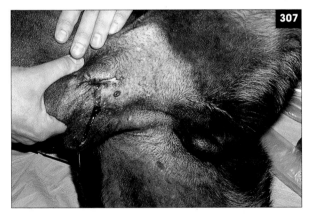

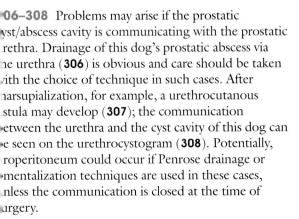

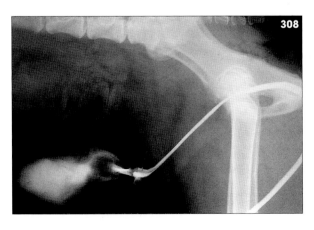

306–308 Problems may arise if the prostatic cyst/abscess cavity is communicating with the prostatic urethra. Drainage of this dog's prostatic abscess via the urethra (**306**) is obvious and care should be taken with the choice of technique in such cases. After marsupialization, for example, a urethrocutanous fistula may develop (**307**); the communication between the urethra and the cyst cavity of this dog can be seen on the urethrocystogram (**308**). Potentially, uroperitoneum could occur if Penrose drainage or omentalization techniques are used in these cases, unless the communication is closed at the time of surgery.

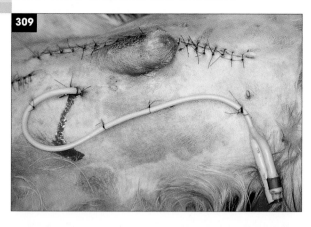

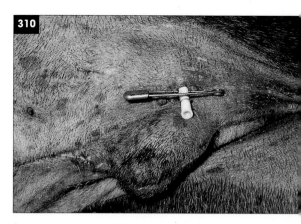

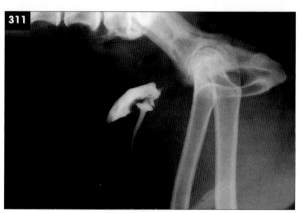

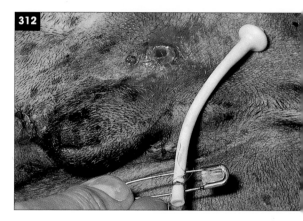

309–312 One possible way of treating a prostatic cyst/abscess that communicates with the urethra and in which the communication cannot be found and closed, is to use tube drainage. Although Foley catheters can be used for this purpose (**309**), mushroom tip catheters (**310**) are better. They are less likely to come out prematurely and the tube can be shortened. If there is local wound swelling, the shortened tube tends to be displaced subcutaneously. This can be prevented by the use of an external flange or, as in this case (**310**), a safety pin (this was padded but is shown just prior to removal). Water-soluble, iodine-based contrast medium can be introduced through the tube from time to time to check the size of the cyst cavity and to determine that the communication with the urethra has closed (**311**) before the tube is removed (**312**).

Of all the techniques used, omentalization ± partial resection (**313–317**) appears to give the best results. A biopsy should always be taken during surgery, since proportion of prostatic cysts and abscesses have carcinoma of the lining (see **117** and **303**). Complications of prostatic cyst/abscess treatment include urethral trauma, peritonitis and uroperitoneum or urethrocutaneous fistulation (if there is communication with the prostatic urethra and depending on which surgical procedure has been performed) (see **306–308**).

Idiopathic prostatic haemorrhage responds to oestrogens, anti-androgens and castration (see **272**, **294**) and probably represents a form of benign disease but without obvious enlargement.

The prostate can become displaced, usually into perineal ruptures (**318**) and sometimes into inguinal hernias or abdominal ruptures. Treatment involves reduction and repair of the hernia/rupture (see **202**, **230**).

Finally, a word of warning. Trauma to the prostate is rare but may be iatrogenic. The most distressing event is when the prostate is inadvertently excised as a complication of cryptorchidectomy. It can also occur when a 'mass' in a perineal rupture is excised and proves to be a displaced prostate gland. The outcome is usually disastrous and euthanasia is required in most cases, with the threat of reporting for professional incompetence.

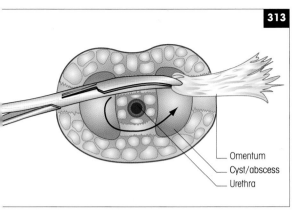

Omentum
Cyst/abscess
Urethra

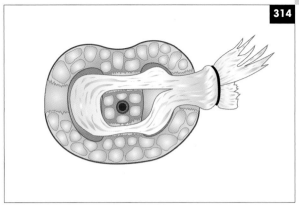

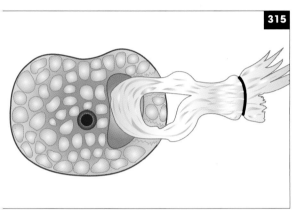

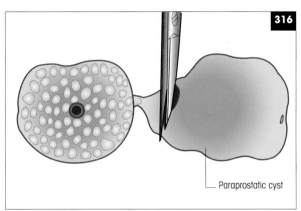

Paraprostatic cyst

nd/or litigation looming. This complication is more likely to happen if cryptorchidectomy is attempted through small laparotomy incisions; therefore, exploration of the abdomen for retained testes should take place through an incision large enough to allow good orientation. Masses in perineal ruptures should not be excised until ultrasonography and/or contrast radiography has revealed what they are.

313–317 Omentalization of prostatic cysts and abscesses gives good results. In the original description of the technique by White and Williams (1995), multiple intraprostatic abscesses were illustrated and the omentum completely encircled the urethra through communications generated between these (**313, 314**). However, if the cyst/abscess cavity is more localized, such encirclement may not be necessary (**315**). In the case of large cysts, partial cyst resection can be performed before omentalization, as described by Bray *et al* (1997) (**316, 317**).

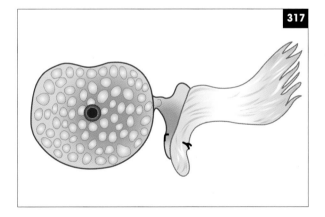

318 Displacement of the prostate and bladder into a perineal rupture. This can be confirmed pre-operatively using ultrasonography and/or urethrocystography (see Chapters 2 and 3).

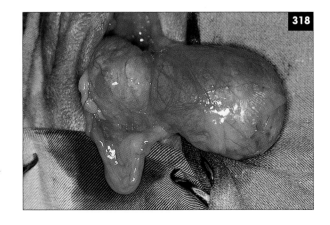

6 Urinary tract trauma

And because I am happy, & dance, & sing, they think they have done me no injury
William Blake (1757–1827)

TRAUMA CAN AFFECT any region of the urinary tract. In order of the incidence in which trauma is diagnosed, these areas are the bladder, urethra, kidney and ureter. However, it is estimated that the kidneys of 25% of small animals in road traffic accidents are traumatized; the fact that these are not diagnosed with the same frequency suggests that most heal spontaneously.

Renal trauma

THE MAIN PROBLEMS associated with renal trauma are blood loss and reduction in renal function, although the latter is only a clinical problem in the rare event of bilateral renal trauma or injury to the kidney(s) of an animal with pre-existing renal disease or which has only one kidney. Depending on the extent of the damage, subcapsular, retroperitoneal and intraperitoneal haemorrhage may occur. Severe cases require supportive intensive care (intravenous plasma expanders, blood) before surgery. In mild cases, conservative treatment is sufficient. Organized subcapsular haematomata are occasionally found incidentally in older cats in which the initial trauma was not noticed by the owners. In severe cases of unilateral renal trauma, nephrectomy may be required. If damage is confined to one renal pole, partial nephrectomy can be performed by stripping the peritoneum and renal capsule from the traumatized portion. Following removal of damaged tissue and ligation of arcuate vessels at the cut surface, the renal capsule and peritoneum are repaired over the site of excision. Haemostasis during surgery is accomplished by digital compression of the renal vessels by an assistant.

There is controversy concerning the total nephrectomy technique (**319–337**). It is suggested that the renal artery and vein should be ligated separately to avoid the risk of an arteriovenous fistula developing. The author has yet to meet anyone who has seen such a fistula and he believes the risk of haemorrhage during dissection and separation of the artery and vein is higher than the risk of arteriovenous fistula; he ligates the vessels as one, first with a proximal simple ligature and then a transfixing ligature distal to that. The second controversy is about whether removal of the ureter is required or not. If the ureter is involved in the disease process or is diseased itself, ureteronephrectomy should be performed. If not (e.g. renal trauma cases), the ureter can be ligated proximally during nephrectomy.

Renal trauma may result in serious intra-abdominal or retroperitoneal haemorrhage, but rarely results in uroperitoneum; lower urinary tract damage is the more usual cause of this.

319–337 Nephrectomy technique.
(**319**) The kidneys can be approached from flank or ventral abdominal incisions. The author prefers a ventral midline abdominal approach, extending from the xiphisternum to just caudal to the umbilicus (for nephrectomy alone) or to the pubis (for ureteronephrectomy). The advantage of the midline approach over a flank approach is that it allows access to a greater area of the abdomen. This is important in cases of renal neoplasia (to examine for the presence or absence of metastases) and/or if the ureter is also diseased and requires removal. In addition, most surgeons are more familiar with this approach than the use of flank incisions. Once the abdomen is opened, the kidneys must be located.
(**320**) The right kidney is found by locating and elevating the duodenum, as illustrated.
(**321**) If the duodenum is now reflected medially, the right kidney is exposed and the mesoduodenum is used to prevent the intestines from returning to the right side of the cranial abdomen.
(**322**) The left kidney is located similarly, except that the descending colon is found and elevated.

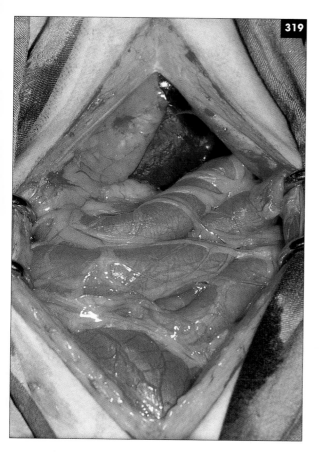

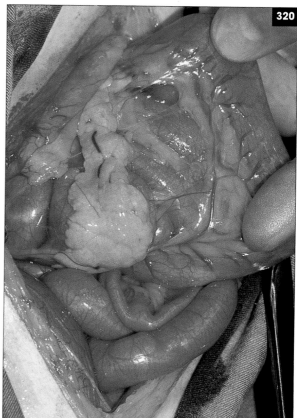

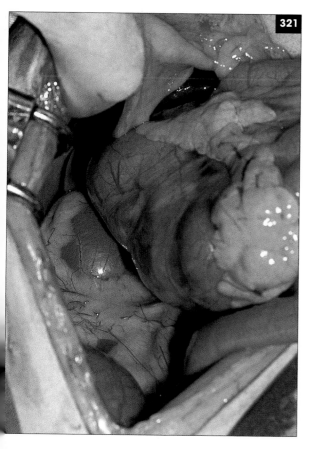

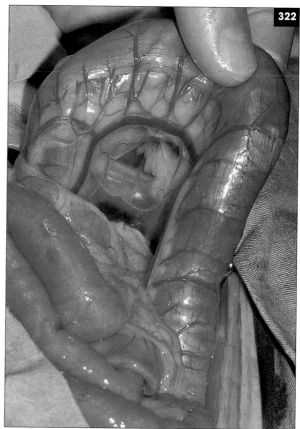

(**323**) The descending colon is reflected medially, the mesocolon retaining the intestines and allowing access to the left kidney. The kidneys are attached to the dorsal abdominal wall by the overlying peritoneum and cannot immediately be raised to the level of the abdominal incision. Access can be improved if an assistant depresses the ipsilateral side of the incision, reducing the distance between incision and kidney.

(**324**) The kidney is gently elevated and the surrounding viscera packed off with moistened swabs. This particular animal has severe chronic pyelonephritis associated with ureteral ectopia.

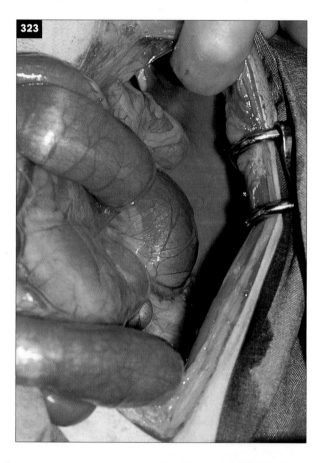

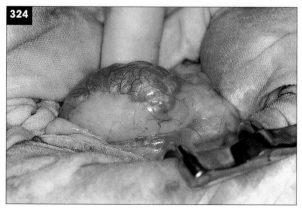

Prolonged tension on the kidney should be avoided because the transference of traction to the renal vessels may result in tension on the major abdominal vessels, particularly the vena cava, reducing venous return of blood to the heart. Any tension placed on the renal hilus during surgery should only be intermittent.

(**325**) The peritoneum overlying the kidney and the hilar fat are freed from the kidney, allowing the renal vessels (cranial to the left in the illustration) and ureter (caudal to the right in the illustration) to be isolated. Once the peritoneum is incised, blunt, finger dissection is the safest way to free these tissues. The peritoneum may be firmly attached to the kidney by the disease process, making separation difficult and resulting in haemorrhage from multiple points on the kidney surface. Such haemorrhage is usually minor and ceases when the renal vessels are ligated. More severe haemorrhage should be controlled by direct application of pressure (it is not usually possible to clamp and ligate vessels, since the bleeding points are often on the surface of the kidney) or local diathermy. Large peritoneal vessels should be ligated. Great care should be taken when dissecting around the hilus to avoid damage to the major renal vessels.

(**326**) Once the kidney, its vessels and proximal ureter are freed from their attachments, the renal vessels are ligated, with the first (simple) ligature placed proximally around both the artery and vein. It has been suggested that the renal artery and vein should be ligated separately to avoid the possibility of postoperative arteriovenous fistulation. However, such fistulation seems more of a theoretical than a practical consideration and, in cases of gross renal enlargement and disease, it would be hazardous to attempt to separate the renal vessels.

(**327**) Once the first ligature has been tied, a transfixing ligature is placed distal to (i.e. the kidney side of) it. The second ligature is transfixed by taking it between the renal artery and vein. If this is not possible, the ligature can be taken through one of these vessels, since haemorrhage is prevented by means of the first, simple ligature and by clamping of the vessels adjacent to the renal hilus.

(**328**) The transfixing ligature is now tied as shown. The material used for ligation is a matter of personal preference; the author prefers to use synthetic absorbable material. It should be noted that such double ligation of the renal vessels is not always possible, particulary if the kidney is grossly enlarged and grossly diseased (see **32, 33** and **378**). In such cases the enlarged kidney and presence of local adhesions may make access to and identification of renal vessels difficult, and sometimes single ligation only is possible.

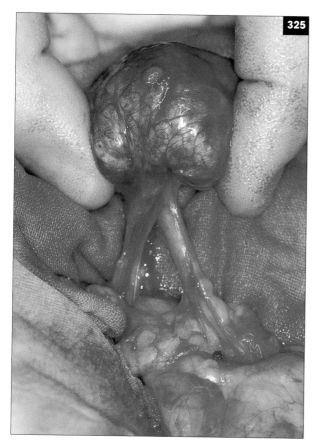

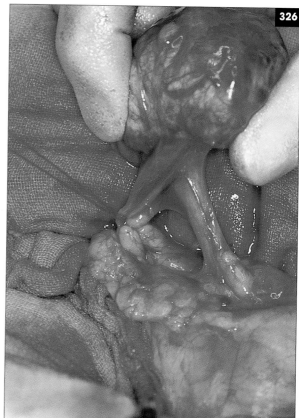

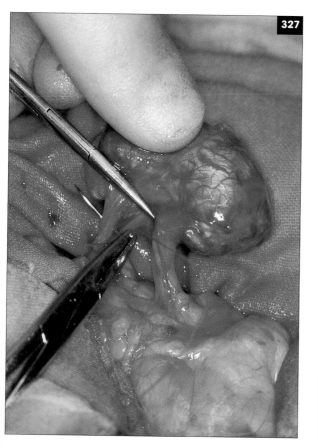

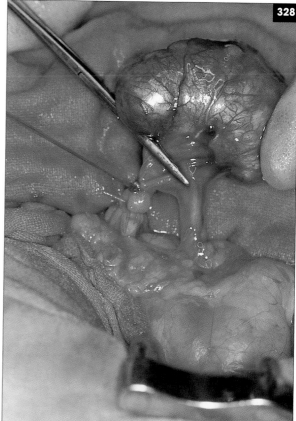

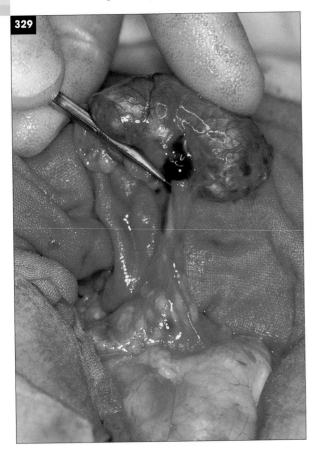

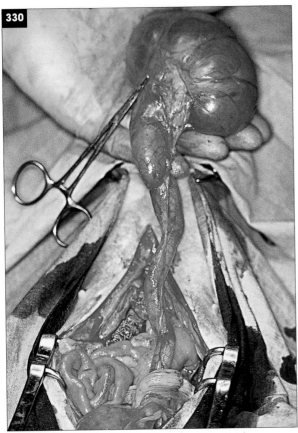

(**329**) With the vessels sectioned between the distal, transfixing ligature and the clamps, only the ureter now remains attached to the kidney. If the ureter is not diseased (as in this case), it can be clamped at the hilus and a simple ligature applied approximately two centimetres distally. The kidney can now be removed by sectioning the ureter between the clamps and ligature. Some authors suggest that the ureter should be excised down to its insertion into the bladder, as otherwise it may act as a reservoir for stagnant urine (especially if vesico-ureteral reflux is present), predisposing to urinary tract infections. However, normal ureteral peristalsis in an undiseased ureter results in ureteral emptying; the author has experienced no difficulties in animals in which healthy ureters have not been excised during nephrectomy.

(**330**) If the ureter is diseased, it should be removed along with the kidney. In this example, both hydro-nephrosis and hydroureter are present. If the ureter is not removed, it may act as a reservoir for urinary tract infections. If gentle traction is applied to the ureter, it can be pulled from its retroperitoneal position. Note, however, that the distal ureter passes beneath the uterine horn and its broad ligament (or vas deferens in the male). There is no need to perform traumatic dissection to the uterus or broad ligament; the distal ureter can be freed as illustrated in **331–337**.

(**331**) The distal ureter is identified (arrowed) as it passes beneath the uterus and broad ligament and inserts into the dorsal wall of the bladder. Caudal is to the left in this photograph.

(**332**) The tip of a pair of artery forceps is passed through the peritoneum and beneath the ureter as it enters the dorsal wall of the bladder (the ureter is viewed from the opposite side in this and subsequent photographs and so caudal is now to the right).

(**333**) The forceps are used to place ligature material beneath the ureter as they are withdrawn.

(**334**) The ureter (and its associated vessels) are ligated adjacent to the bladder wall, clamped approximately one centimetre cranially and sectioned between the clamps and ligature.

(**335**) The freed, distal ureter is now ligated as shown to prevent urine leakage following removal of the clamps.

(**336**) The ureter cranial to the uterus is now grasped and gentle cranial traction applied.

(**337**) The distal ureter can be pulled retroperitoneally below the uterus and broad ligament (or vas deferens in the male) until it is completely freed. The kidney and ureter can now be removed from the abdomen. The stumps of the renal vessels are checked for the absence of bleeding before the abdomen is closed routinely.

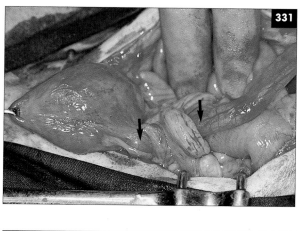

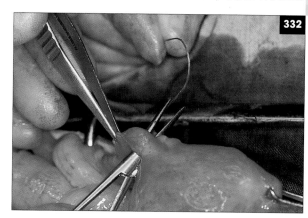

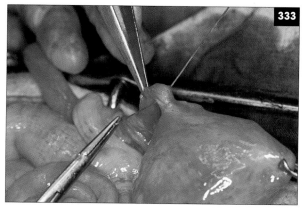

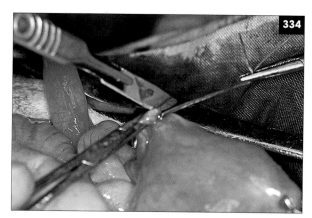

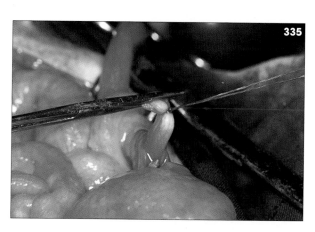

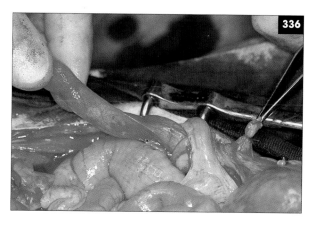

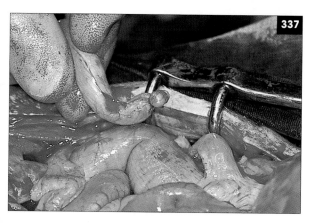

Uroperitoneum

In order of incidence, bladder, urethral or ureteral rupture may occur. Initially, at least, the ruptured ureter or urethra may leak retroperitoneally, delaying the metabolic effects of urine leakage (urea and potassium and hydrogen ions are absorbed much more slowly from the retroperitoneum than they are from the peritoneal cavity). In animals with rupture of the urinary organs and uroperitoneum, the metabolic disorders of uraemia, acidosis and hyperkalaemia are life-threatening and must be corrected before surgery. Intravenous fluids (initially without potassium) and sodium bicarbonate, coupled with peritoneal drainage and dialysis (or lavage), are most useful. Alternatively, insulin and glucose can be administered to drive the potassium ions back into the cells. In addition, an indwelling urinary catheter is helpful, particularly in cases of bladder rupture (**338, 339**), to minimize further urine leakage into the abdominal cavity.

338–339 Ruptured bladder management.
(**338**) This Flat-coated Retriever has a ruptured bladder; the urethrocystogram is illustrated in **77**. The dog is not sedated, but rather it is collapsed due to the metabolic consequences of uroperitoneum (i.e. hyperkalaemia, acidosis and azotaemia). The effects of the acidosis and hyperkalaemia on the heart can be appreciated from the ECG (**339**). An over-the-needle intravenous cannula has been inserted just caudal to the umbilicus and is being used both to drain urine from and to introduce dialysing fluids into the peritoneal cavity.
In this example, abdominocentesis is being used (along with intravenous fluid therapy and the insertion of an indwelling urethral catheter) to relieve the uroperitoneum and its metabolic consequences. Although syringe suction may speed the rate of fluid removal, it is frequently counterproductive, since omentum or other abdominal viscera may be sucked onto the end of the drain/catheter, preventing the exit of fluids. It is often better to allow the fluid to drain passively through the drain/catheter.

Treatment of urinary tract trauma

Gross renal trauma usually results in haemoperitoneum rather than uroperitoneum and has previously been discussed in this chapter. Repair of the ruptured bladder involves debridement (**340**) followed by repair of the defect (see **151–160**).

Mild cases of urethral trauma may respond to the use of an indwelling urethral catheter (see **89–91**) or tube cystostomy (see **231–234**) as a urinary bypass in order to allow healing, but severe urethral ruptures should be treated surgically. Such cases may have the same metabolic problems as animals with bladder rupture (although these may be more insidious in onset if leakage is initially into the retroperitoneum), which must be corrected before surgical intervention.

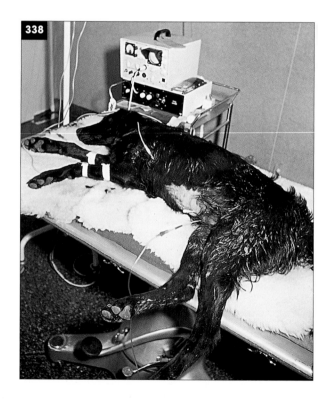

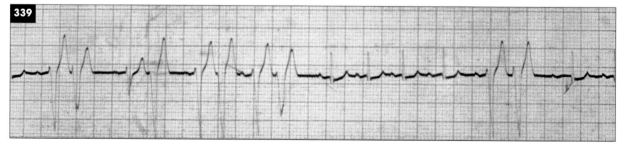

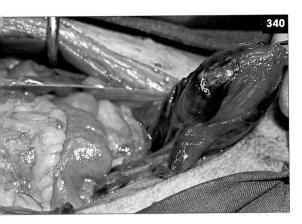

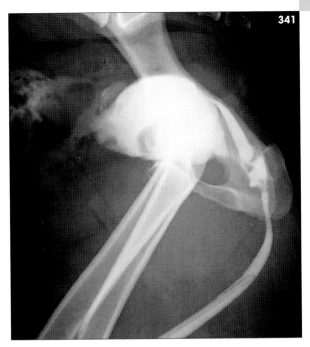

However, it can be hard to determine the exact extent of the tear. Contrast radiography may define the location of the defect but rarely its size, making the decision to bypass or surgically repair difficult (**341, 342**). If in doubt, it is better to explore the area surgically. There are, sometimes, poor results in animals with severe rupture using bypass alone, especially if the rupture continues to leak (**343–348**). Urine in the retroperitoneum leads to severe necrosis (**343–350**). The tube cystostomies illustrated in **232–234** and **343, 344** were used to treat animals with urethral trauma. In the case of the cat in **232–234**, surgical repair was required after the urethra failed to heal, and the dog in **343** and **344** developed an inoperable urethral stricture and had to be euthanased.

340 Rupture of the dorsal wall of the bladder in an Irish Setter bitch after a road traffic accident. Note the devitalized tissue, which should be debrided before repair of the defect. Bladder repair in these cases should be deferred until the patient is stabilized (see **338, 339**).

341, 342 Lateral (**341**) and ventrodorsal (**342**) radiographs illustrating rupture of the urethra in a male Springer Spaniel after a road traffic accident. The pelvic fracture just caudal to the right acetabulum is fairly innocuous, but the urethra is damaged in two sites. The retrograde positive contrast urethrogram shows damage to the urethra just proximal to the ischial arch, and the accumulation of contrast medium within the pelvic cavity is due to contrast medium leaking retroperitoneally and around the prostate before entering the peritoneal cavity. At surgery, the pelvic urethra was found to have completely torn away from the caudal prostatic urethra. This was treated by repair of the urethral transection and urinary bypass using a urethral catheter (see also **351, 352**).

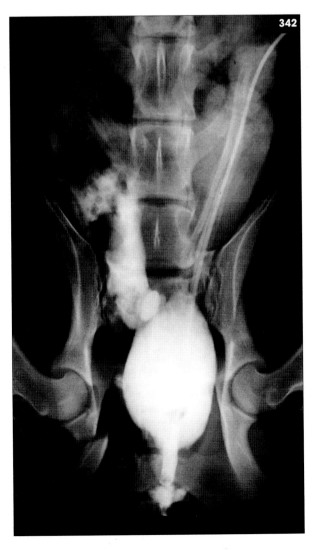

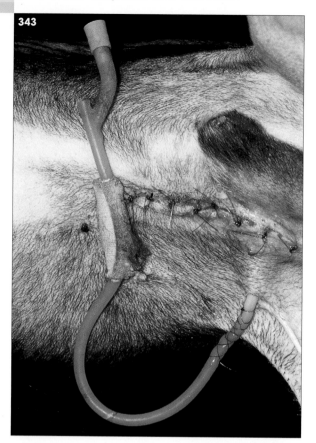

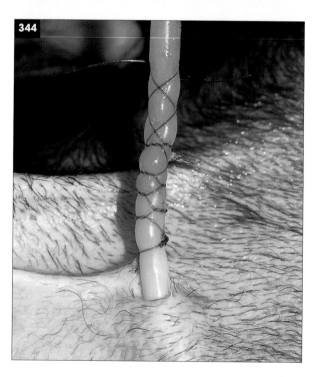

343, 344 A Foley catheter has been used for tube cystostomy in this dog with a urethral rupture to provide urinary bypass (**343**). The catheter has been secured using a Chinese finger trap suture (**344**). The photograph was taken at the time of catheter removal after two weeks. Although the urethra healed, the dog was dysuric due to urethral stricture at the site of the rupture and periurethral fibrosis of intrapelvic soft tissues after urine-induced necrosis.

345–348 (**345**) Attempts to treat a urethral rupture in a cat using tube cystostomy with a Jackson's catheter. Note the early perineal necrosis associated with the necrotizing effects of leaked urine.
(**346**) Further necrosis, including the anus, occurred in this cat.
(**347**) The cat was dyschezic and faecal passage was obstructed within the pelvis.
(**348**) A barium enema revealed this to be due to complete rectal obstruction resulting from rectal necrosis and fibrosis. This cat was euthanased.

349 The necrotizing effect of urine can be seen in this Dachshund with a rupture of the pelvic urethra. Sloughing of intrapelvic tissues and perineal skin has occurred. This was treated as an open wound until the defect was filled with healthy granulation tissue and then primary skin closure was performed (see also **355, 356**).

350 Identification of the site of urethral rupture during surgery can be difficult because of leakage of urine into surrounding soft tissues. Pre-operative contrast radiography is essential to allow a planned surgical approach and to minimize trauma to the area. In this bitch, contrast radiography had demonstrated a tear in the proximal urethra close to the neck of the bladder. This enabled repair to be performed without the need for pubic osteotomy, although the animal's progress meant that this technique had to be performed later (see **359, 360**). The discolouration of the perivesical fat is due to infiltration by urine.

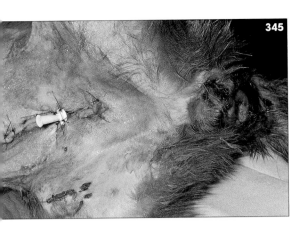

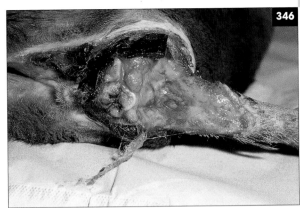

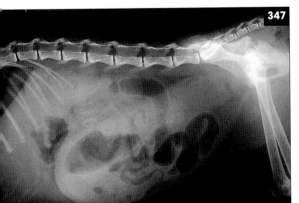

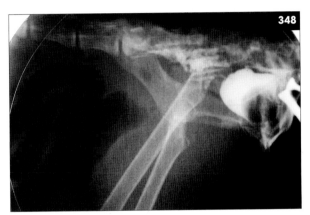

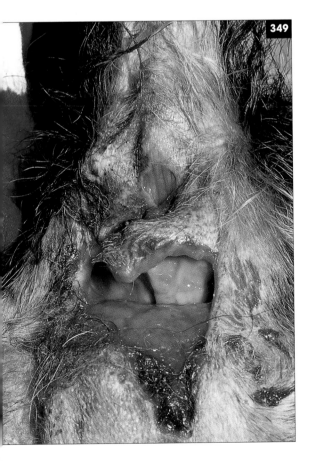

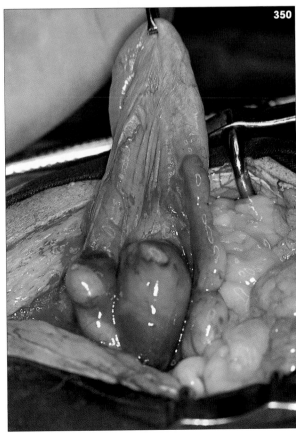

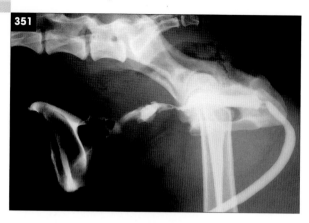

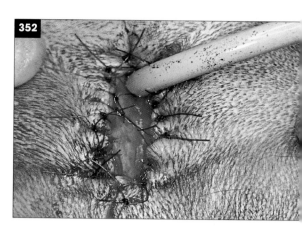

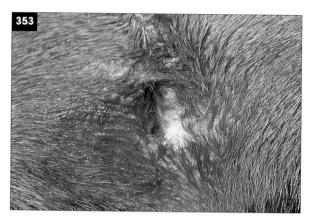

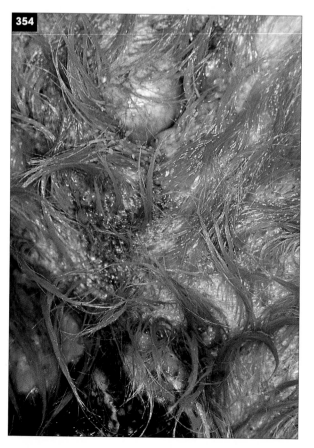

Urethral repair (especially intrapelvic) is difficult and splitting of the pubis may be required to facilitate exposure. An indwelling catheter should be used as a urethral 'splint' postoperatively. Long-term problems with urethral ruptures include strictures (**351–354**, **359–364**), possibly as a result of inadequate tissue debridement before repair (**355, 356**).

351, 352 (**351**) Follow-up retrograde positive contrast urethrogram in the dog in **341** and **342**, two months after urethral repair. The dog is dysuric due to urethral strictures at the sites of previous urethral damage and repair (the caudal and cranial pelvic urethra). Urethral stricture is a common complication of urethral trauma. This dog was treated by dilation of the strictures via a perineal urethrostomy and the use of a 22Fr Foley catheter during healing (**352**). This dog subsequently did well. Perineal urethrostomies can be used to bypass untreatable, more distal urethral injuries or obstructions, but they are associated with long-term problems in some dogs (see **353, 354**).

353, 354 Perineal urethrostomy may result in urinary tract infection and skin scalding. A perineal urethrostomy stoma in a Doberman Pinscher five years after surgery is shown (**353**). Apart from minor dampness of the hairs around the stoma after urination, this animal has experienced no ill effects. At the other extreme, the Golden Retriever illustrated (**354**) (also five years after perineal urethrostomy) has serious chronic problems. The skin around the perineal stoma is scalded and the scrotum is ulcerated. Struvite crystals can be seen attached to the hairs around the stoma and are associated with chronic, recurring cystitis associated with infection by *Proteus* spp.

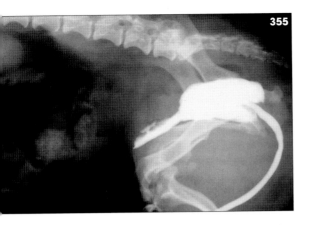

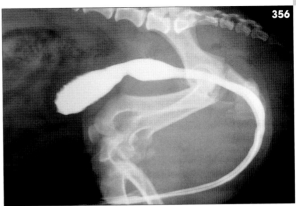

355, 356 The author is convinced that part of the cause of urethral strictures after repair is inadequate debridement of the torn ends of urethra before suturing. Devitalized urethral tissues may remain after repair, leading to breakdown of the repair and/or secondary intention rather than primary wound healing. These radiographs were taken at the time this Dachshund was presented after a road traffic accident (**355**) and two weeks after surgical repair (**356**). The pelvic urethra of this dog was virtually transected, with less than a quarter of the urethral circumference remaining intact. Urine-induced tissue necrosis affected the intrapelvic tissues and perineal skin (see **349**). A pubic osteotomy provided good exposure of the urethral tear and the torn edges of urethra were debrided back to healthy tissue before repair (this meant resecting up to 1 cm of urethra from each edge). As the follow-up radiograph shows, the urethra has healed in a normal anatomical configuration without stricture formation.

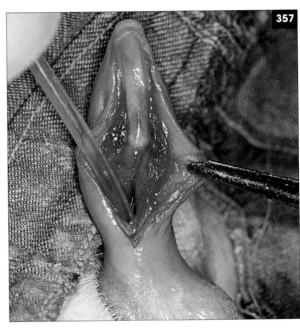

357, 358 Urethrostomy should be performed as distally as possible.
(**357**) This male cross-bred is dysuric due to a stricture of the terminal penile urethra associated with previous urolithiasis at that site (which is unusual). This is treated by extending the ventral part of the external urethral orifice caudally. A ventral midline incision is made in the urethra from the external urethal orifice to proximal to the stricture using Metzenbaum scissors. A urinary catheter has been placed in the urethra proximal to the stricture. The granulation tissue responsible for the urethral narrowing can be seen in the terminal penile urethra.
(**358**) The penile integument is now sutured to the urethral urothelium, as shown, using a simple continuous pattern of synthetic absorbable material (in this case, 3/0 polyglactin). In effect, this creates a large external urethral orifice which extends distal to the site of obstruction, thus relieving the dysuria.

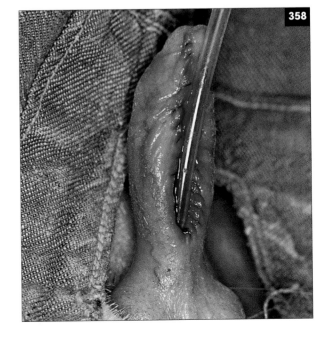

If strictures are severe, they can be bypassed (if distal) by means of more proximal urethrostomies (see **180**, **187–199** and **357–358**). Intrapelvic strictures can sometimes be resected (**359–364**).

In animals with gross, irreparable intrapelvic urethral trauma, it is possible to perform a prepubic urethrostomy (**365–367**) but postoperative scalding of the ventral abdomen with urine, incontinence and stoma stricture may occur and the long-term results are disappointing and often unacceptable to the owner.

Ureteral tears are difficult to locate and IVU is a useful pre-operative diagnostic aid (**368**). During surgery it may be necessary to perform a ventral cystotomy and catheterize the affected ureter (a 3Fr catheter is suitable for most dogs). The ureter can then be detected in its retroperitoneal position and the site of leakage demonstrated by retrograde infusion of sterile saline via the catheter (**369**). Following repair (using 4/0 or 5/0 synthetic absorbable material), the catheter is left *in situ* as a splint for 1–3 days. Distally, the catheter is passed out via the bladder and urethra, and sutured to the vulva or prepuce. Follow-up contrast radiography is useful to determine the progress of healing (**370–372**).

359, 360 Contrast radiographic (**359**) and urethroscopic (**360**) appearance of a urethral stricture resulting from urethral trauma and repair in the Cavalier King Charles Spaniel bitch in **350**. Urothelial polypoid masses, such as the one illustrated just distal to the stricture in **360**, are not uncommonly found in the urethra after trauma.

361–364 (**361**) A pubic osteotomy has been performed on the bitch illustrated in **359, 360**. The bladder is in the bottom right of the picture and the pelvic fat and fascia ventral to the urethra have been separated in order to locate the urethral stricture (the lower forceps are pointing to the stricture). (**362**) The strictured length of urethra is resected and a urinary catheter inserted through the external urethral orifice and across the gap between the cut ends of urethra into the proximal urethra and bladder. Bleeding urethral vessels are clamped at the levels of the cut urethral ends, as shown, and subsequently ligated. Initially, it is useful to leave the vascular clamps on the vessels, since this facilitates orientation of the urethra, thus preventing rotation of one urethral segment relative to the other during repair. (**363**) The first two sutures (in this case, 3/0 polyglactin) are placed 180° apart in the lateral walls of the urethra. This facilitates subsequent suture placement and, if the ends of these sutures are left long, as shown, they can be used to rotate the urethra during placement of sutures in the dorsal urethral wall. (**364**) Suturing is continued around the circumference of the urethra until the urethral ends are joined. Sutures should be placed close together (approximately 2 mm apart) and tied tight enough to achieve apposition without crushing the urethral tissues. Once suturing is completed, the pubic osteotomy and ventral, caudal laparotomy are closed routinely. The catheter can be left *in situ* as an indwelling catheter for urinary bypass for 7–10 days.

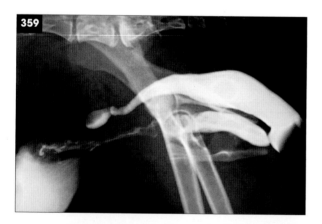

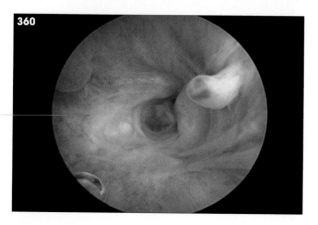

365–367 (**365**) Prepubic urethrostomy. In this example, irreparable membranous urethral damage occurred when the cat was shot; the air gun pellet entry hole can be seen on the caudal right thigh. A tube cystostomy had been performed for urinary bypass. The photograph was taken ten days after a prepubic urethrostomy. (**366**) A close-up view of the area. The urethra cranial to the damaged area has been transected, tunnelled through the caudal abdominal wall, spatulated and sutured to the prepubic skin to form a stoma (arrowed).

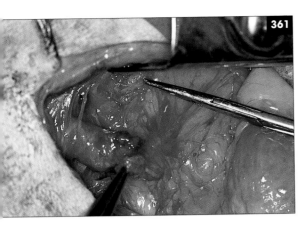

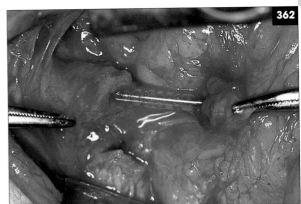

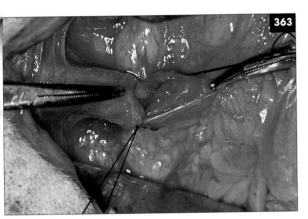

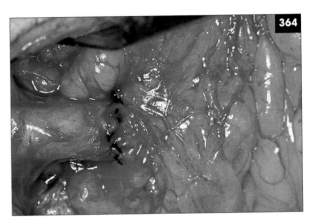

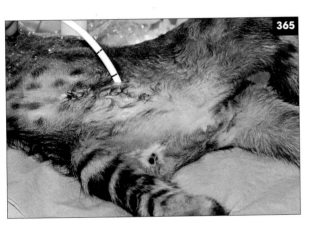

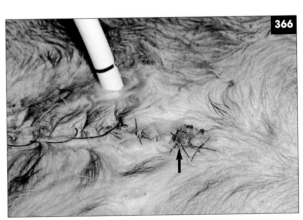

(**367**) The long-term results of this procedure may be disappointing. In this cat (a different animal from that shown in **365** and **366**), urine leakage and skin scalding are chronic postoperative problems, although they were tolerated by this particular owner.

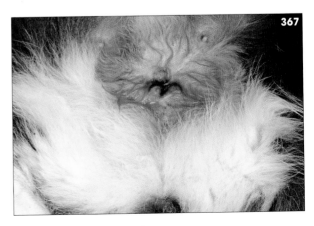

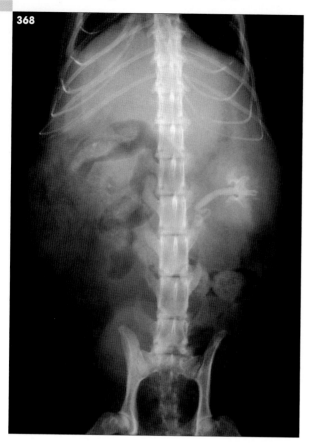

Ureteral tears in cats are extremely difficult to repair even with an operating microscope, because of the small size of the ureter, and ureteronephrectomy may be required in such cases (**368**). The author has no experience of tube nephrostomies as ureteral bypass procedures.

It should also be remembered that urinary tract trauma may be iatrogenic (see **127, 128** and **373–375**).

368 Proximal ureteral rupture in a cat after a road traffic accident, demonstrated by IVU. Note the increase in soft tissue density surrounding the left kidney due to retroperitoneal leakage of urine. Ureteronephrectomy was performed in this cat.

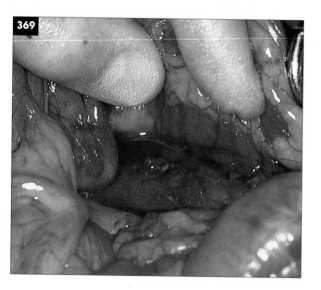

369 The laparotomy appearance of a ruptured ureter in the Golden Retriever bitch illustrated in **34**. Urine can be seen leaking from the retroperitoneal tissues, the swelling of which (due to infiltration of urine and cellulitis) prevents visualization of the ureter. Retrograde ureteral catheterization was used in this case to facilitate identification of the ureter and the tear during dissections through the swollen peri-ureteral tissues. In fact, the urolithiasis, which led to the rupture, was associated with bilateral ureteral ectopia, and the right ureter was transplanted into the bladder after repair.

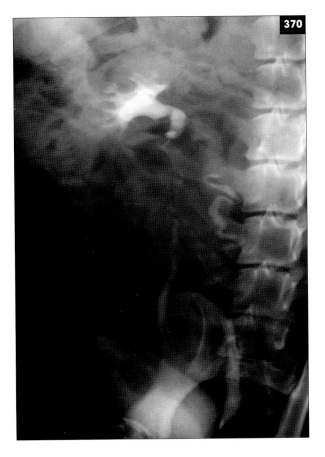

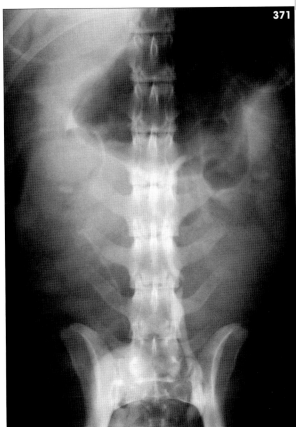

370–372 (**370**) A follow-up radiograph (IVU) taken four days after repair of the ruptured ureter illustrated in **34** and **369**. Renal pelvic dilatation is still apparent and the site of repair appears narrowed. When the IVU was repeated six weeks postoperatively (at the time of transplantation of the second ureter), the renal pelvis and ureter had returned to normal sizes (**371, 372**). The renal calculi (struvite) had dissolved after elimination of the associated urinary tract infection.

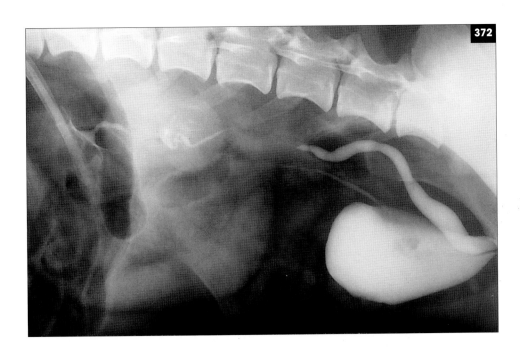

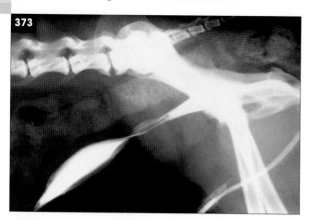

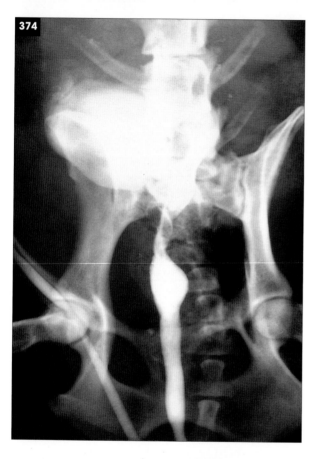

373, 374 Lateral (**373**) and ventrodorsal (**374**) urethrocystograms illustrating 180° iatrogenic bladder torsion. This was produced during cystopexy in a male dog with perineal rupture, and resulted in dysuria.

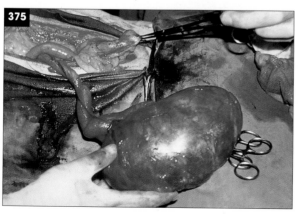

375 Gross hydro-ureter and hydronephrosis resulting from adhesion of the ureter to the linea alba after ovariohysterectomy. It is difficult to imagine how this could have been produced. Most trauma to the ureter during ovariohysterectomy is usually associated with ligation of the uterine/cervical stump and results in a ureterovaginal or, rarely, vesicovaginal fistula rather than uroperitoneum (see **441–449**).

As must have rung the harvest-song of Linos, of bloody water in a heap of stones
Allen Tate (1899–1979)

As MENTIONED IN the previous chapter, trauma to the urinary system may result in haematuria. In this chapter, other causes of haematuria are described.

Animals with frank blood in the urine are often presented as emergencies by their owners. In most cases urgent treatment is not required, but exceptions are animals with severe blood loss, trauma or infection. Once again, it is the pre-operative supportive care of these animals that is most important.

Haematuria may be associated with a vast array of conditions. In general terms haematuria may occur as a result of:

- Urolithiasis.
- Urogenital
  - inflammation/infection.
  - neoplasia.
  - trauma.
- Idiopathic renal haemorrhage.
- Prostatic disease.
- Urethral prolapse.

Many of these conditions are discussed elsewhere in this book, so the diagnosis and treatment of only the remainder will be described.

Diagnosis

THERE ARE TWO main questions to answer:
- Where is the haemorrhage coming from?
- What is the haemorrhage due to?

The history often suggests if the bleeding is from the lower or upper urinary tract. Animals with macroscopic lower urinary tract bleeding usually have other lower urinary tract signs such as dysuria, pollakiuria, nocturia and incontinence, whereas these are usually absent in upper urinary tract bleeding. The cause of the haemorrhage is more difficult to determine and usually requires contrast radiographic, ultrasonographic and laboratory examinations aimed at the area of the urinary tract suggested by the history. For example, if the dog has other lower urinary tract signs, lower urinary tract radiographic and ultrasonographic studies are usually performed first. Bacteriological examination should also include antibiotic sensitivity testing in cases where there is infection.

If renal calculi (**376**) are detected, it should be determined that they alone are responsible for the haematuria before they are treated (see **16** and **377**). Kidney stones are sometimes detected incidentally on radiographs of clinically normal dogs, but beware big nipples; they may be mistaken for nephroliths on ventrodorsal films if they overlie the kidneys (see **17**, **18**).

376 Renal calculus (struvite) removed from a Labrador Retriever bitch. The calculus conforms to the shape of the renal pelvis, with the 'beak' corresponding to the proximal ureteral orifice.

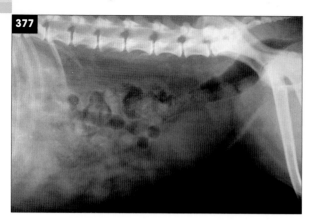

377 Lateral abdominal radiograph of the Cavalier King Charles Spaniel in **16**, made four months later. This dog had been presented with severe, acute abdominal pain. Abdominal radiography revealed renal and vesical calculi (see **16**), which were assumed to be the cause of the signs. However, blood laboratory analyses revealed that the pain was associated with acute pancreatitis for which the animal was treated with prophyllactic antibiotics (ampicillin) and a bland diet (chicken and rice). This radiograph reveals that all the calculi have disappeared. This animal had triple phosphate crystals and bacteria in its urine; presumably the calculi were of the same material and dissolved in response to elimination of urinary tract infection and a high biological value, low-protein diet. This case underlines two points: the renal calculus or calculi may not be responsible for the presenting signs, and nephrotomy may not be required to eliminate them (see also **370–372**).

Bladder and urethral neoplasia have been described in Chapter 4. The commonest kidney tumour in small animals is renal lymphosarcoma in the cat. In affected cats there may be other evidence of leukaemia/lymphosarcoma such as lymph node enlargement and positive FeLV testing. Renal neoplasia is rare in the dog. The commonest primary canine renal tumour is the carcinoma (**378**), but the clinical signs may be non-specific. For example, gross haematuria may be absent unless the neoplasm is a haemangiosarcoma (**379**), and the renal tumour may be detected as a craniodorsal abdominal mass in a dog being examined for weight loss. Sometimes, the detection of lung metastases is the first indication that an animal has a primary renal tumour so, if lung metastases are detected in an animal with no obvious primary tumour, the kidneys should be examined carefully. Animals with renal carcinoma may have polycythaemia. Thoracic and abdominal radiography (including IVU), ultrasonography, urine and blood laboratory examinations and, possibly, scintigraphy are required to check for metastases and assess the presence and function of the other kidney if surgery is contemplated, as well as for diagnosis. If available other modalities such as MRI/CT scanning are extremely useful.

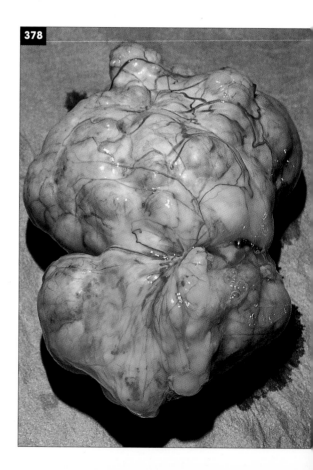

378 Renal carcinoma excised from a German Shepherd Dog. Unusually, this dog did well after surgery (most carcinomas of this size are associated with local and distant metastatic disease; this was absent in this case). Location and double ligation of the renal vessels during nephrectomy (see **319–337**) in cases such as this is more challenging.

Laparotomy, biopsy or excision and pathology may be required for a definitive diagnosis in some instances, though, if available, ultrasound-guided biopsies are useful to indicate if surgery is likely to be worthwhile (see **118, 119**). During laparotomy, the abdominal cavity should be examined for tumour spread, especially to the local renal lymph node and blood vessels. Invasion of renal vasculature or the vena cava, for example, makes the prognosis poorer (because of the likelihood of intravascular seeding of malignant cells) and the surgery more difficult if not impossible. Other primary kidney tumours in the dog are lymphosarcomas, haemangiomas (or sarcomas) (**379**) and nephroblastomas (**380, 381**). It should also be borne in mind that the kidney is a common site for metastases of non-renal tumours to develop and that neoplasia of pararenal organs (e.g. adrenal gland) may spread to involve the kidneys.

Two interesting conditions are prostatic haemorrhage and idiopathic renal haemorrhage. The former leads to blood loss via the urethra between micturitions and is diagnosed on this history and the elimination of other causes of haematuria and prostatic bleeding (see Chapter 5). Blood loss in cases of idiopathic renal haemorrhage can be severe (**382**) and the main differential diagnosis is renal haemangiosarcoma (**379**).

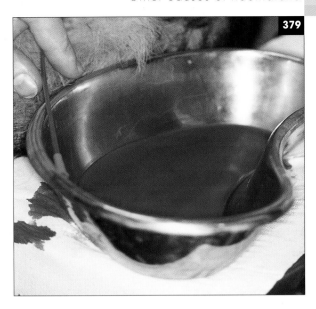

379 Severe haematuria in a German Shepherd Dog with a renal haemangiosarcoma. Despite the severity of the haematuria, these tumours may be quite small and difficult to detect.

380, 381 (**380**) Renal tumour demonstrated ultrasonographically in an adult Golden Retriever bitch. The tumour is obstructing the renal pelvis, resulting in hydronephrosis. The accummulation of urine in the renal pelvis improves the ultrasonographic contrast, enhancing demonstration of the hilar mass. (**381**) The excised kidney (sectioned sagittally). This proved to be a nephroblastoma. The section of tumour from the right half of the kidney has been removed to demonstrate the secondary hydro-nephrosis that was present. Ectopic nephroblastomas can occasionally occur in the spinal cord.

382 Severe haematuria in a Labrador Retriever with idiopathic renal haemorrhage. This can mimic the level of haematuria found in cases of renal haemangiosarcoma (see **379**).

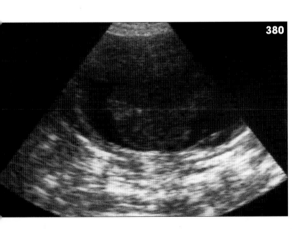

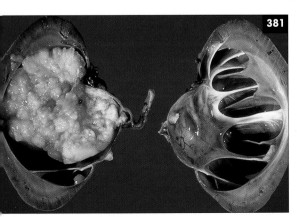

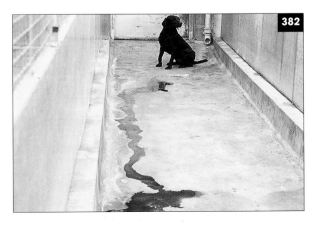

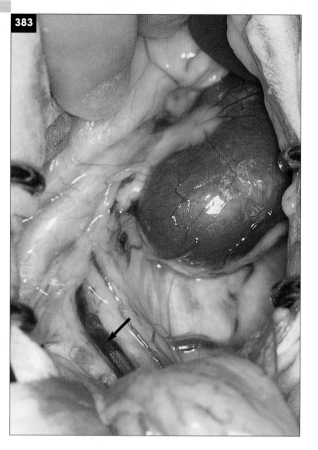

Earlier reports suggested that this problem was confined to young animals and was only unilateral. While this is mainly the case, the author has also seen the condition in mature dogs and as a bilateral condition. Previously (after all other investigations were inconclusive), the diagnosis relied on demonstration of renal haemorrhage by ureteral visualization (383–385) and catheterization during cystoscopy or cystotomy (386, 387). The kidney was then removed in case an undiagnosed neoplasm was present, and idiopathic haemorrhage was only confirmed when histopathology revealed no abnormalities apart from the bleeding (388, 389). The increased availability of ultrasonography in veterinary practice, coupled with contrast radiographic and laboratory examinations means that veterinary surgeons can be more confident that this is not a neoplastic condition and avoid unnecessary laparotomies. Nowadays, therefore, unless the dog is becoming anaemic from the renal bleeding, most cases are treated by benign neglect after reassuring the owners that this is not a malignant condition. Occasionally, the bleeding will resolve spontaneously. It is prudent to perform haematology on these dogs on a regular basis to ensure that anaemia is not developing, since this would be an indication for nephrectomy.

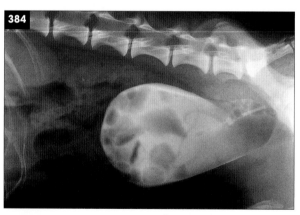

383–385 (**383**) In cases of renal haemorrhage, the ureter (arrowed) may be visualized at laparotomy, filled with blood and resembling a blood vessel, but this is unusual. The condition is intermittent in many animals and any investigations, including exploratory laparotomy, are a waste of time unless performed on a day when haematuria is present.
(**384**) The blood clots entering the bladder from the ureters are often vermiform, as are some of the clots in this dog's bladder, and they may be seen on contrast cystography.
(**385**) Sometimes, the vermiform clots are passed by the dog.

386, 387 Diagnosis is usually made by ureteral catheterization via a ventral cystotomy (**386**) and urine sampling from each ureter (**387**). If bleeding is unilateral, nephrectomy may be required to prevent further blood loss if the dog is becoming anaemic. The excised kidney should be submitted for histopathological examination; idiopathic renal haemorrhage can only be diagnosed by eliminating other possible diagnoses on pathological examination.

388, 389 The excised kidneys from two dogs with idiopathic renal haemorrhage.

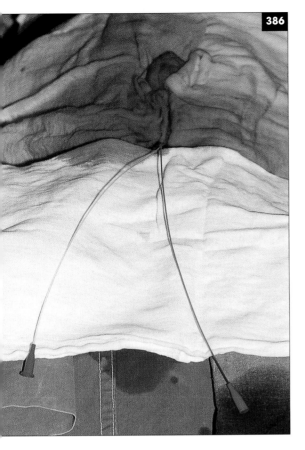

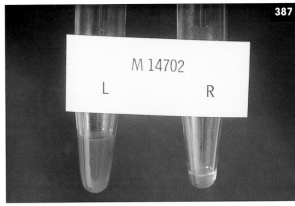

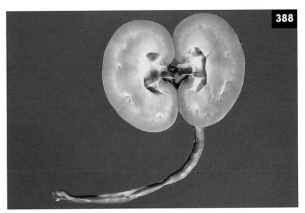

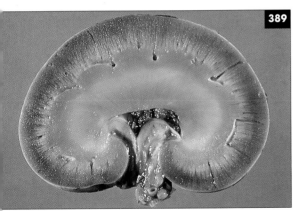

Urethral prolapse usually results from excessive masturbation. It appears as a 'red pea' on the tip of the penis (**390**) and results in blood dripping from the prepuce, especially when the dog is (sexually) excited. This may be confused with haematuria (by the owners) and has to be differentiated from prostatic disease. Examination of the penis is diagnostic.

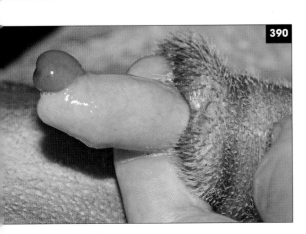

390 Urethral prolapse in a seven-month-old Bull Mastiff. The prolapse appears as a 'red pea' on the tip of the penis. During surgery, the prepuce can be retracted and the penis supported by the use of a bandage, loosely tied around the base of the penis and pulled caudally (see **6**).

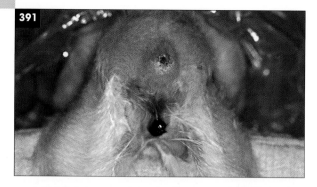

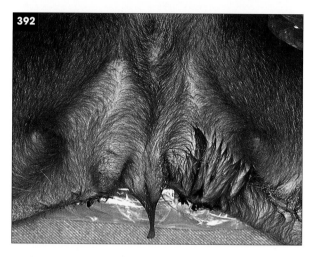

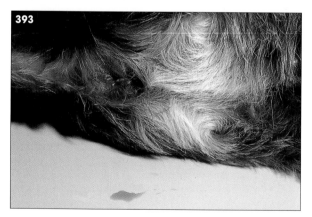

Treatment

U<small>RINARY TRACT INFECTION</small> should be treated wit[h]
intensive antibiotic therapy based on bacteriologic
sensitivities for a period of at least four weeks, unle[ss]
the antimicrobial manufacturer's recommendation
for a shorter period of treatment. Any disorders tha[t]
may be predisposing to urinary tract infection shoul[d]
be corrected (**391–397**). Response should be assesse[d]
by repeating urine cultures. Bladder calculi may requi[re]
surgical removal (**398**); non-responding cases of diph[-]
theritic cystitis may require debridement of dea[d]
bladder mucosa (**399, 400**); severe pyelonephrit[is]
(if confined to one kidney) may necessitate nephre[c]
tomy (**319–337**); and prostatitis may respond to th[e]
use of appropriate antibiotics and castration (se[e]
Chapter 5).

391–395 Congenital recto-urethral (illustrated in a
cat [**391**]) or rectovaginal fistulae (shown in a Vizla
puppy [**392**]) usually present as cases of dyschezia,
since anal atresia is usually also present. These cases
carry a guarded to poor prognosis if atresia ani is
present. In the absence of atresia ani, affected animals
may be presented because of recurring urinary tract
infection secondary to contamination of the lower
urinary tract by faecal organisms. The dog illustrated
in **393** is leaking urine from the rectum, especially
during micturition, and it also has cystitis. A catheter
has been passed *per rectum* into the fistula and on into
the bladder (**394**). This facilitates identification of the
fistula for ligation during surgery (**395**). The prognosis in cases uncomplicated by atresia ani is good.

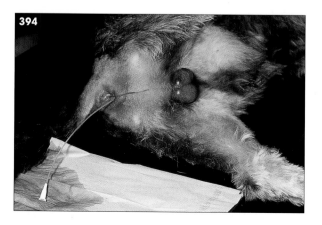

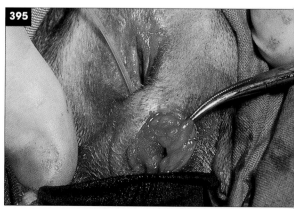

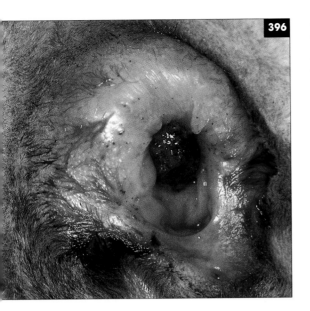

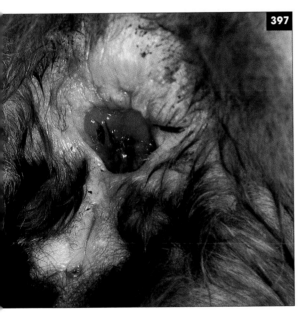

399, 400 Occasionally, chronic, localized cystitis fails to respond to antibiotic therapy and it may be necessary to debride ulcerated, necrotic and/or diphtheritic urothelium before healing can take place. Cystotomy in this Great Dane bitch with chronic haematuria has revealed the nature of a urothelial lesion (**399**) detected on double contrast cystography. The infected, necrotic urothelium was excised (**400**) and the bitch made an uneventful recovery. It is important that any excised tissues are submitted for histopathological and bacteriological examination to determine the exact nature of the disease process and obtain a prognosis.

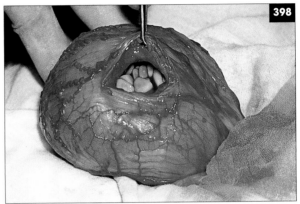

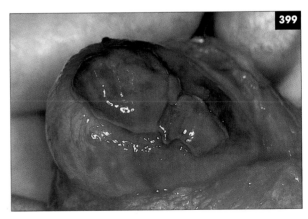

396, 397 Contamination of the lower urogenital tract with faecal organisms can also occur in cases of congenital anovaginal cleft, as in this juvenile Persian cat (**396**). This is treated using a reconstructive technique to give the cat a perineum (**397**). The cases illustrated in **391–395** and **396, 397** are rarely encountered in general practice and so are best referred for treatment.

398 Bladder calculi can be removed via a cystotomy. Older texts describe a dorsal cystotomy for this procedure, but there is no advantage over a ventral cystotomy. An alternative approach would be to attempt calculus dissolution, but in male dogs there is the potential risk that small calculi remnants may pass into the urethra and cause obstruction.

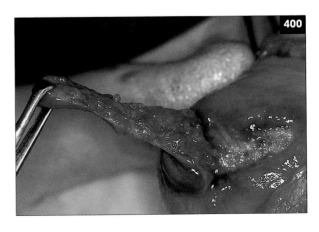

Nephrotomy to treat renal calculi (**401–403**) is this author's last resort and he rarely performs this surgery nowadays, preferring dietary dissolution if possible. Nephrotomy is reserved for animals in which dietary dissolution has failed, the calculi appear to be the main cause of the animal's signs and there is no evidence of renal failure. All other cases are treated or managed medically. In the author's experience, renal calculi are often an indication of a chronic renal problem and not the main cause of the animal's symptoms *per se*. Great care should be taken to assess renal function pre-operatively since, in animals in compensating renal failure, nephrotomy may precipitate an acute crisis (**404**).

If no metastases are detected and the contralateral kidney is functioning well, nephrectomy of a neoplastic kidney may be performed (see **319–337** and **378, 380, 381**), but (depending on the tumour type) the prognosis is usually guarded to poor, although some animals do well after surgery.

Cases of prostatic haemorrhage usually respond well to castration (see Chapter 5) and nephrectomy is indicated when idiopathic renal haemorrhage is present and resulting in severe blood loss (see **382–389**).

401–403 (**401**) During nephrotomy, the kidney is approached and located as illustrated in **319–337**. It is essential that intravenous fluids are started pre-operatively and that whole blood or plasma expanders are to hand in case of unexpected intra-operative haemorrhage. In the author's opinion, nephrotomy (like nephrectomy) requires the help of a surgical assistant. The assistant grasps the hilus of the kidney between the thumb and index finger of one (gloved) hand and uses the other hand to depress the ipsilateral side of the abdominal incision to improve access to the kidney by the surgeon. As well as supporting the kidney for surgery, the assistant can feel the pulse in the renal artery through the perihilar peritoneum and fat and can thus occlude the renal vessels during surgery (for haemostasis). Similarly, pressure on the hilus will occlude the ureter, preventing fragments of the calculus from passing into the ureter during surgical manipulations. The alternatives to the use of an assistant's finger and thumb involve dissecting through the perihilar tissues, isolating the renal vessels and occluding them temporarily with atraumatic vascular clamps or loops. Using an assistant is quicker, easier and less traumatic, and there is no need to move the kidney during surgery if it is desirable to resume renal blood flow; the assistant merely relaxes his/her grip slightly. An incision is made through the peritoneum, renal capsule and renal parenchyma into the renal pelvis. The location of the renal pelvis can be appreciated when the scalpel blade contacts the calculus. The size of the incision is related to that of the calculus, but usually extends approximately over the middle third of the greater curvature of the kidney.

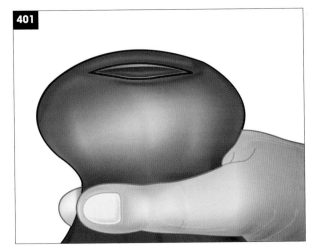

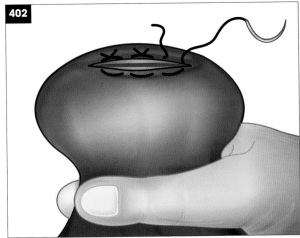

the calculus is removed using forceps and submitted for analysis. Any remaining fragments of calculus are removed with forceps and by flushing the renal pelvis with sterile saline. If the surgery thus far has taken more than ten minutes, the assistant should allow blood to flow through the kidney for a minute or so. Haemorrhage from the nephrotomy can be reduced by gently holding the incision closed during this period.

402) The nephrotomy incision is closed by apposing the renal parenchyma using horizontal mattress sutures of synthetic absorbable material. The sutures should be placed through the peritoneum, renal capsule and renal cortex, but they should not be placed too deep or too tight in order to avoid damage to the arcuate vessels at the corticomedullary junction. They should be placed to a depth approximately half that of the renal cortex.

403) After apposition of the renal parenchyma, the renal capsule and peritoneum are closed in a single layer using a simple continuous suture, again of synthetic absorbable material. The abdomen is closed routinely. Some authors compromise between the technique described here and non-suturing methods by closing only the renal capsule and peritoneum.

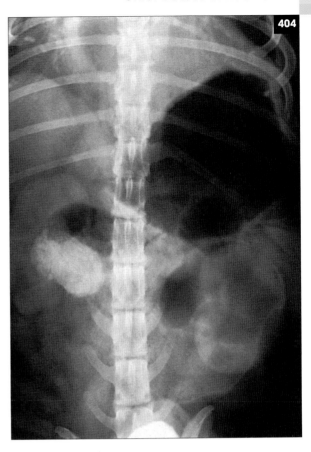

404 Ventrodorsal nephrogram during IVU on an 11-year-old debilitated Pug with chronic haematuria. A large renal calculus is present in the right renal pelvis. However, note also the irregular outline of both kidneys and the poor renal opacification by contrast medium. This animal had severe, chronic, bilateral pyelonephritis, and nephrotomy to remove the calculus was sufficient to induce acute, fatal renal failure. This case illustrates the potential hazards of nephrotomy and the need for good laboratory work-up before surgery is considered. This case would have been better managed medically.

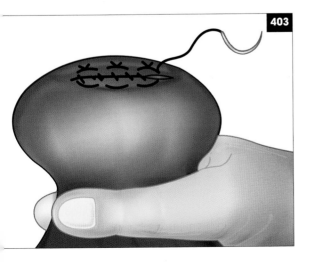

Although prolapse reduction and purse-string suturing of the external urethral orifice have been used to attempt to treat urethral prolapse, they are not to be recommended, and the best form of treatment is prolapse amputation (**405–410**), after which the dog is sedated for 5–7 days to prevent excitement and erections (and thus more bleeding) during healing of the area. Recently, prolapse reduction and full-thickness sutures placed into the urethral lumen to prevent recurrence have been used successfully to treat this condition. The dog's oversexuality should also be treated to prevent recurrence.

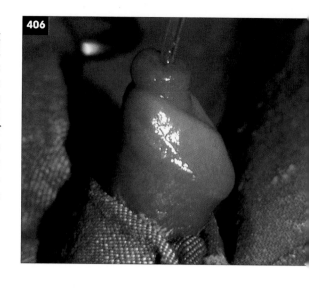

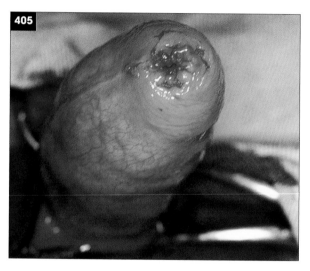

405 The risk of postoperative stricture during urethral prolapse amputation can be reduced by attention to suturing. This is the immediate postoperative appearance of the penis of the dog shown in **6**. The urethral urothelium has been sutured to the penile integument using simple interrupted sutures of 5/0 polyglactin placed closely together. If a continuous pattern is used, it should not be used unbroken around the whole circumference of the repair (**406–410**); if the sutures are pulled too tight, a purse-string suture may result, leading to stenosis.

406–410 (**406**) To improve access during urethral prolapse amputation, the penile urethra is catheterized and the penis elevated (as shown in **6**). The penis is prepared for aseptic surgery using dilute antiseptics followed by sterile saline and avoiding the use of concentrated solutions and irritants such as surgical spirit.
(**407**) The prolapse is elevated and the penile integument incised at the base of the prolapse. The incision is continued through the urethral urothelium to expose the catheter in the urethral lumen.
(**408**) The urethral urothelium and penile integument are apposed using fine synthetic absorbable sutures. A simple interrupted pattern or continuous suture (as shown) can be used. If a continuous pattern is used, it is advisable to place the suture over a third of the circumference, tie it and then use two further, separate continuous sutures to complete the remainder of the repair in order to reduce the risk of stenosis.
(**409**) Once the incised section is sutured, a further section is incised around the circumference of the base of the prolapse and the urethral urothelium and penile integument apposed as described in **408**. Eventually, the prolapse will be attached to the penis by only a small section of tissue, as shown.
(**410**) The final section of tissue is sectioned and the prolapse removed. The remaining defect is closed by apposition of the urethral urothelium and penile integument. The remaining suture ends are cut short after tying. Note the oozing haemorrhage that occurs. This is not serious, but it may persist as a postoperative problem and alarm and/or inconvenience the owners if they are not made aware of its possibility. Postoperative haemorrhage can be minimized by prevention of trauma to the surgical site and treatment of the dog's excitement, especially if sexual.

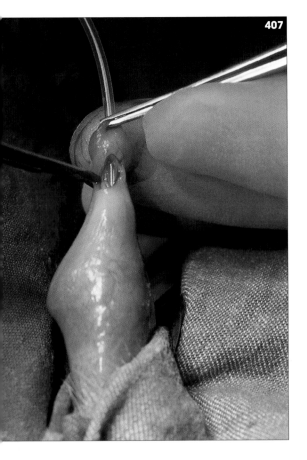

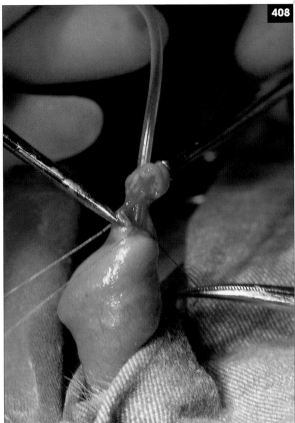

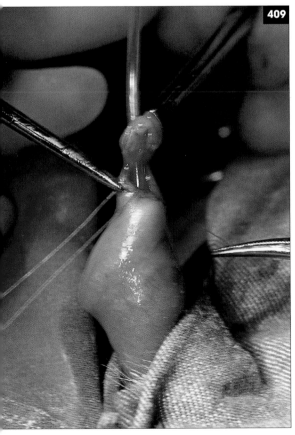

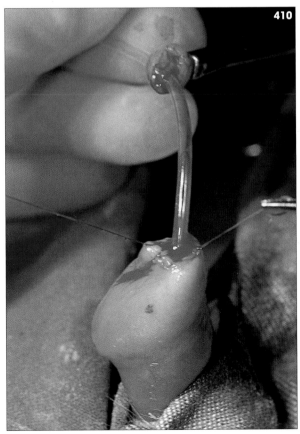

8 Urinary incontinence

O Geordie, Jingling Geordie, it was grand to hear Baby Charles laying down the guilt of dissimulation, and Steenie lecturing on the turpitude of incontinence.
Sir Walter Scott (1771–1832)

I will incontinently drown myself
William Shakespeare (1564–1616)

ANIMALS WITH URINARY incontinence are presented either as juveniles with congenital causes or as adults with acquired causes of incontinence. These two groups are dealt with separately. The pathophysiology and treatment of the commonest cause of urinary incontinence, urethral sphincter mechanism incompetence, are areas where most progress has been made over the past 25 years. This is described in more detail at the end of this chapter.

Urinary incontinence in juvenile animals

In juvenile animals, urinary incontinence may be associated with:
- Ureteral ectopia.
- Congenital urethral sphincter mechanism incompetence.
- Bladder hypoplasia.
- Pervious urachus.
- Intersexuality.
- Congenital neurological conditions.

Ureteral ectopia

THIS IS MAINLY a problem of dogs (but is also reported in cats, horses and cattle). The cause is unknown but hereditary factors and vitamin imbalance in the dam may play a role. In the UK, Labrador and Golden Retrievers (see **3**) and Skye Terriers are at risk for this condition. The condition is much commoner in bitches than in male dogs. The condition may present later in life in male dogs; it is possible that the stronger male urethral sphincter mechanism allows male dogs to cope with this problem without leakage until it deteriorates.

There is a species difference in that most canine ectopic ureters run an intramural route through the bladder wall, whereas those of cats are usually extramural to the bladder wall (**411, 412**). Incontinence may be continuous (see **3**) or intermittent and, even in bilateral cases, normal micturition usually occurs. Diagnosis is by contrast radiography (see **31** and **53**) and/or ultrasonography, when a dilated intramural ureter (an ureterocoele) may be detected (see **235, 236,**). Most ectopic ureters terminate in the urethra (in the male dog, they all terminate in the prostatic urethra); sometimes, they terminate in the vagina. Contrary to earlier opinion, there is no relationship between the side and the termination of ectopic ureters.

Treatment in dogs usually involves stomatizing (**413–425**) or, in cats, transplanting (**426, 427**) the ureter into the bladder. It is vital that any pre-existing urinary tract infection is eliminated before stomatization or transplantation. Excision of the ureter and associated kidney is required if severe secondary disease is present (see **32, 33** and **319–337**). The average veterinary surgeon in general practice will only see one case of ureteral ectopia in approximately five years, and so these cases are best referred.

411, 412 Ureteral ectopia in the dog and cat. Note that in the dog (**411**) the ectopic ureter usually enters the bladder wall at the normal site, but travels intramurally, beyond the trigone and bladder neck, to open ectopically (arrowed), in this case into the distal urethra. In the cat (**412**) the ectopic ureter completely bypasses the bladder. This cat also has a congenital failure of the müllerian ducts to fuse, and so the body of the uterus and vagina are absent, the uteri opening individually into the vestibule.

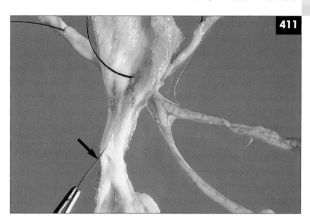

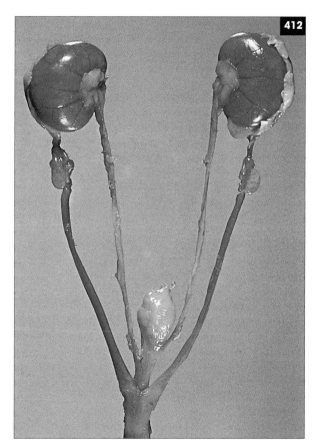

413, 414 Diagrams summarizing the stomatization technique used to treat an intramural ectopic ureter (**413**). The ureter is stomatized into the bladder at the level of the trigone and ligated just distal to the stoma (**414**). The technique is described in detail in **415–425**, although these cases are best referred.

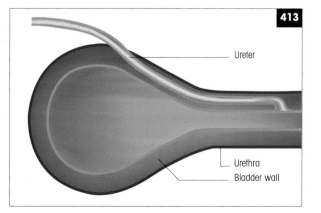

Ureter

Urethra
Bladder wall

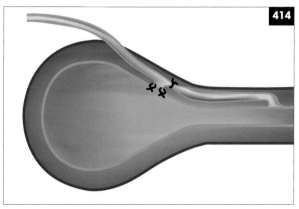

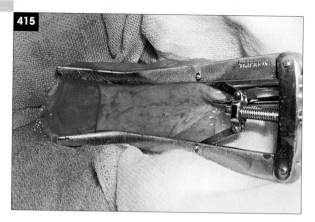

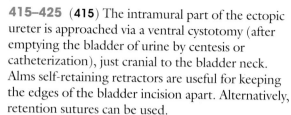

415–425 (**415**) The intramural part of the ectopic ureter is approached via a ventral cystotomy (after emptying the bladder of urine by centesis or catheterization), just cranial to the bladder neck. Alms self-retaining retractors are useful for keeping the edges of the bladder incision apart. Alternatively, retention sutures can be used.

(**416**) The urothelium of the dorsal bladder wall is incised over the intramural ureter at the level of the trigone. If the ureter is dilated (e.g. as in **429**), the site of incision is easy to identify, but difficulty may be encountered in identifying the location of intramural ureters of normal size. Applying pressure to the bladder neck may result in retention of urine in the ureter and facilitate identification, as may passage of a small (3 or 4Fr) urinary catheter up the ectopic ureter from its termination, if possible.

(**417**) The ureter is then located within the bladder wall. It is usually much paler in colour than the bladder wall tissues and feels firmer when grasped with forceps.

(**418**) A ligature is passed around the ureter using synthetic absorbable ligature material.

(**419**) Gentle traction is applied to the ligature in a caudal direction. This supports the ureter while the ureter is incised.

(**420**) A 3 or 4Fr catheter can be passed cranially into the ureter through the incision to facilitate identification of the ureteral stoma and to divert urine from the surgical site. Note the ooze of blood from small suburothelial vessels; although not serious, this makes visualization difficult and necessitates frequent swabbing.

(**421**) The edges of the stoma in the ureteral wall are anastomosed to the edges of the bladder urothelial incision using simple interrupted sutures of fine, synthetic absorbable suture material; the author prefers to use 5/0 polyglactin. Suturing is greatly facilitated and the degree of surgical trauma reduced by the use of fine ocular instruments.

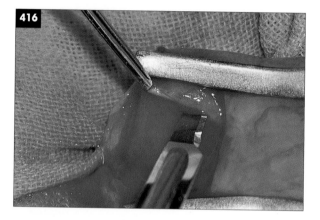

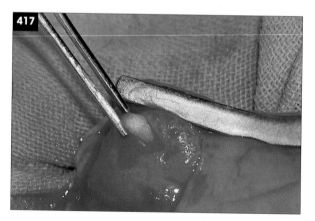

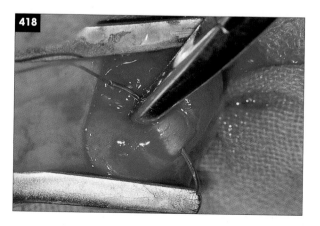

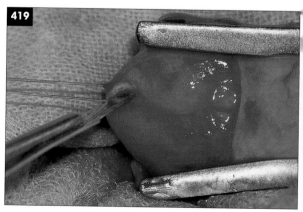

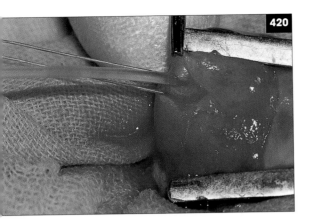

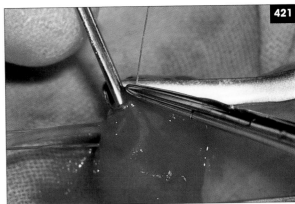

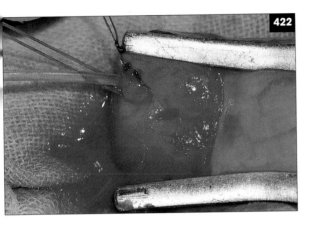

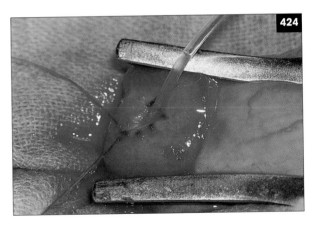

(**422**) Suturing is continued along one edge of the stoma.

(**423**) Once stomatization of the ureter into the bladder lumen has been completed by anastomosis of the ureteral and bladder urothelial incisions, the ligature is tied just caudal to the stoma. In an attempt to prevent recannalization after surgery, some authors double ligate the ureter at this point and section it between the ligatures. However, this involves further dissection close to the bladder neck and may increase the risk of postoperative swelling and bladder neck obstruction.

(**424**) The catheter is removed from the proximal ureter and used to confirm that the ureter distal to the stoma has been occluded by the ligature.

(**425**) The knot of the ligature is buried within the bladder wall by suturing the bladder urothelium over it with a further suture of 5/0 polyglactin. The ventral bladder incision is then closed routinely (see **151–160**).

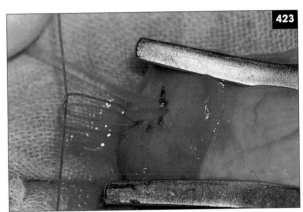

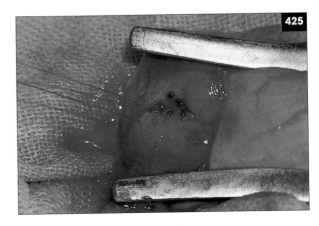

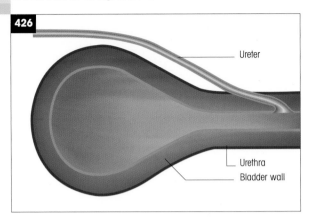

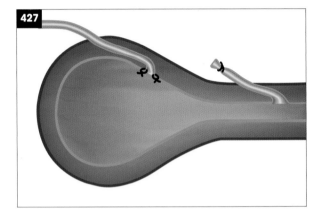

Approximately 50% of animals are completely cured and, in most of the remainder, the incontinence is markedly reduced. A few animals show no improvement after surgery, possibly due to undiagnosed bilateral ectopia, recannalization of the ectopic portion of the ureter after stomatization, concomitant urethral sphincter mechanism incompetence (**428**) anomalous ureteric branches (**429**) or bladder hypoplasia (**430**).

Some authors believe that the intramural ectopic ureter remnant within the urethral wall may adversely affect sphincter function, leading to a poor result and advocating excision. This author remains to be convinced and avoids this because of the risk of postoperative urethral stricture leading to dysuria.

428 This vagino-urethrogram demonstrates that, as well as having an ectopic ureter, the urethra of this five-month-old Golden Retriever is very short and wide. Incontinence in this dog may be complicated by congenital urethral sphincter mechanism incompetence.

429 Distal ureteral branches have been reported as a cause of persistence of urinary incontinence after ureteral transplantation using tunnelling techniques. In these cases the distal ureter opens ectopically, but also communicates with the bladder lumen. Thus, following transplantation using a tunnelling technique, urine may pass from the bladder into the ureteral remnant and exit distally from the termination of the ectopic ureter, bypassing part of the urethral sphincter mechanism and leading to persistence of the incontinence. While such branches may be congenital, they may also be acquired if a ureterocele ruptures into the bladder. A case of bilateral ureteral ectopia is illustrated. A ventral, caudal cystotomy has been performed revealing a dilated intramural ureter (uppermost).

426, 427 Diagrams summarizing the tunnelling technique used to transplant a ureter that completely bypasses the bladder (**426**). The ureter is ligated, transected and tunnelled through the bladder wall (**427**). Its terminal opening is then stomatized into the bladder. This procedure is rarely performed, except in cats or in dogs in which the intramural ureter cannot be found during attempted intravesical stomatization.

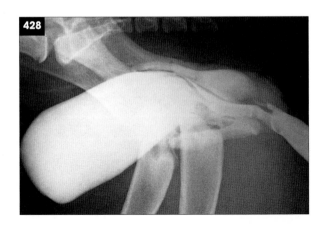

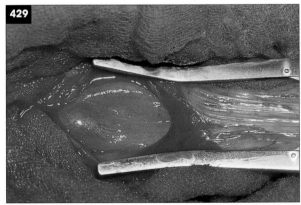

Note the appearance of the second (lowermost) ectopic ureterocele, which is separated from the bladder by only a thin layer of tissue. This ruptured as soon as the overlying tissue was grasped with fine rat-toothed forceps. Rupture of a ureterocele into the bladder lumen may result in so-called distal ureteral branches. The potential problem of distal ureteral branches is overcome if a stomatization technique is used; all that is required is ligation of the intramural ureter distal to its opening into the bladder.

Congenital urethral sphincter mechanism incompetence

DETAILS ARE PROVIDED on this condition under 'Urethral sphincter mechanism incompetence' (see p. 145).

Bladder hypoplasia

A DIAGNOSIS of 'bladder hypoplasia' assumes that we know what bladder 'normoplasia' means, and we do not. There is no information about bladder sizes and their variations in normal animals of different sizes, breeds or ages. It is likely that we are talking about failure of normal bladder development. All bladders begin small and increase in size as the animal grows and produces more urine. In some young animals this does not happen, possibly as a result of insufficient stimulation by increasing urine volumes. This is, therefore, not uncommonly associated with other congenital causes of incontinence (430), but some juvenile animals rarely appear to have a (subjectively) small bladder in the absence of other abnormalities. The diagnosis is confirmed by contrast radiography; only a small amount of contrast medium is required to fill the bladder during retrograde techniques (431). It is important to eliminate other causes of incontinence that may also be present. Treatment of this condition is unsatisfactory. In some animals, following treatment of a concomitant cause of incontinence (e.g. ectopic ureter), the bladder will develop to a normal size. In theory, anticholinergic drugs should help the small bladder to develop by allowing it to fill more before a micturition response occurs, but their efficacy has not been adequately evaluated.

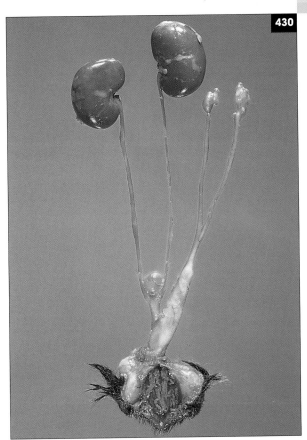

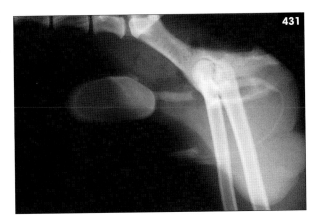

430 Postmortem appearance of a juvenile bitch with ureteral ectopia and congenital urethral sphincter mechanism incompetence. The bladder is very small. Although this is often termed 'bladder hypoplasia', it is more likely to represent a failure of normal development because of the small amount of urine entering and remaining in the bladder during storage. The severe vestibulitis is associated with the continuous incontinence in this dog.

431 'Bladder hypoplasia' demonstrated by retrograde positive contrast urethrocystography in a juvenile male Italian Greyhound with congenital urethral sphincter mechanism incompetence.

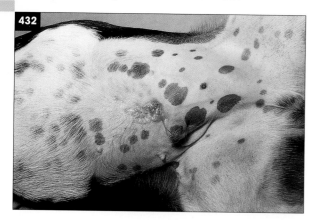

Pervious urachus

THIS CONDITION IS easily diagnosed, since incontinence occurs through the umbilicus, which may be scalded with urine (**432**). Contrast cystography confirms the diagnosis. Treatment involves excision of the urachus (**433**) and repair of the resulting cranial bladder wall defect.

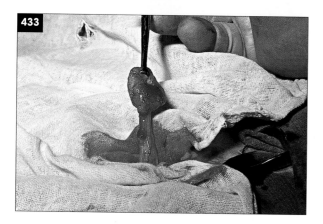

432, 433 Pervious urachus in a Basset Hound puppy. This is rare in small animals (compared with horses and farm animals). Affected animals show urinary incontinence through the umbilicus, with urine scalding of the surrounding skin (**432**). This is treated by excision of the umbilicus and urachus (**433**), followed by repair of the resulting cranial bladder wall defect (see **151–160**) and routine abdominal wall and skin closure.

Intersexuality

RARELY, INTERSEX ANIMALS may be incontinent. There are a variety of anatomical abnormalities that may result in incontinence in intersex animals; the commonest is illustrated (**434**). Diagnosis relies on contrast radiography (**435**). Treatment involves excision of the vagina, uterus and gonads (**436**) via a laparotomy, taking care to preserve the blood and nerve supply to the bladder.

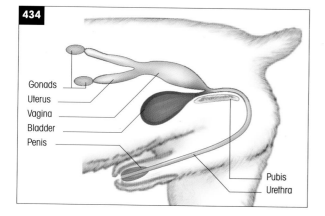

Gonads
Uterus
Vagina
Bladder
Penis

Pubis
Urethra

434 The commonest anatomical abnormality in intersex dogs, resulting in urinary incontinence. This animal has an apparent male urethra (although this may be short and the os penis absent), but has female internal genitalia, the vagina of which opens into the pelvic urethra. During micturition, urine passes from the urethra into the vagina. Leakage of urine from this vaginal reservoir between micturitions results in the sign of incontinence. The gonads can be ovaries, testes or ovotestes, and sex chromosome abnormalities may also be present.

435 Retrograde positive contrast urethrocystography is a good way of demonstrating the abnormalities illustrated in **434**. The vagina (V) is filling retrograde from the pelvic urethra.

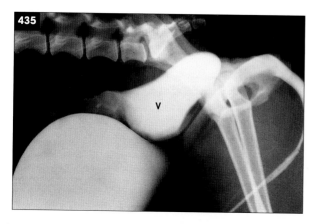

V

436 The excised internal genitalia from an incontinent intersex German Shepherd Dog. In this case the gonads were testes. Great care has to be taken when dissecting the vagina free of its peritoneal covering to preserve the blood and nerves supplies to the urethra and bladder in order to avoid postoperative loss of lower urinary tract function. Note also the presence of struvite uroliths in the lumena of the uteri associated with infection of urine stagnating in the genital tract.

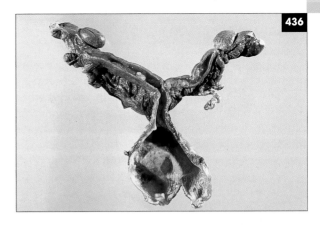

Congenital neurological conditions

THESE INCLUDE MYELODYSPLASIAS, spina bifida and hemivertebrae. Affected animals usually present as obvious neurological cases (e.g. paraparetic). However, some animals may have reasonable ambulation, but faecal and urinary incontinence may be present; this is more likely if an LMN lesion is present (**437, 438**). LMN lesions result in interruption of the sacral reflex arc. Thus, reflex bladder contraction and urethral relaxation do not occur and urine is retained in the bladder, with overflow incontinence. As well as locomotory disturbances, UMN lesions result in spasticity of the external urethral sphincter muscle. Increased urethral resistance leads to urinary retention with overflow incontinence.

Spinal radiography and MRI scanning may confirm the diagnosis. The prognosis for most of these puppies or kittens is poor and euthanasia of the animal is usually required. It is rare for even a dedicated owner to be able to cope with the lifelong need for regular bladder expression and enemas for the animal and, even if this is possible, it raises quality of life issues for the dog/cat.

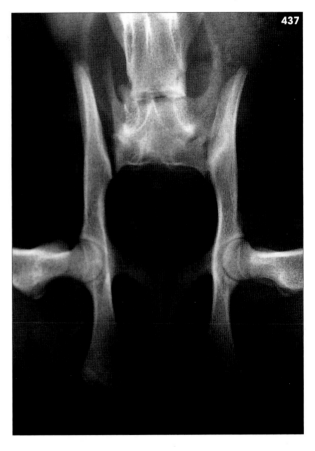

437 Ventrodorsal pelvic radiograph of a juvenile Manx cat that had exhibited urinary and faecal retention and incontinence since birth. Myelodysplasia (abnormal development of the spinal cord) may be accompanied by vertebral spinal abnormalities, which can be detected radiographically. However, radiography itself is not always diagnostic, since many normal Manx cats have this radiographic appearance. Pathological changes (hydromyelia, syringomyelia, meningocele, demyelination and neuronal necrosis) occur in the lumbosacral region and so the condition follows the pattern of LMN disease.

438 Spina bifida in the lumbosacral region of a kitten with LMN signs. The neurological changes are irreversible and, in its severest form, this results in a myelomeningocele.

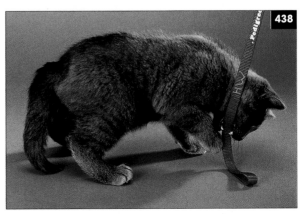

Urinary incontinence in adult animals

CAUSES OF ACQUIRED URINARY incontinence in adult dogs are listed below. Rarely, a congenital abnormality may also result in incontinence, which develops when the dog is adult; for example, some dogs with ureteral ectopia may not exhibit signs as a puppy if the ectopic ureter opens proximally in the urethra and there is a competent sphincter mechanism distal to that.

- Acquired urethral sphincter mechanism incompetence.
- Prostatic disease.
- Bladder/urethral neoplasia.
- Uretero- or vesicovaginal fistula.
- Acquired neurological conditions.
- Overflow incontinence associated with chronic retention.
- Detrusor overactivity/hyperactivity/instability.

Many of these conditions have been discussed in previous chapters of this book (since they result in signs other than incontinence) and so only those features relevant to urinary incontinence will be mentioned in this section.

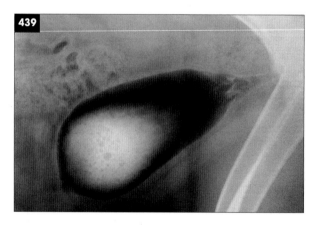

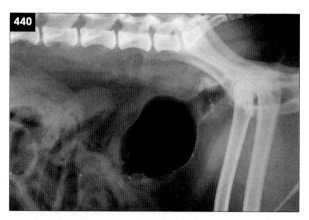

Acquired urethral sphincter mechanism incompetence

See below (p. 150).

Prostatic disease

ALTHOUGH HAEMATURIA and dysuria are the mos common presenting signs, nearly a quarter of dog referred to the author with prostatic disease were sai by their owners to be incontinent. In more than half of these cases, prostatic haemorrhage had been mistake for incontinence of bloody urine (see **5**), but tru incontinence, with or without urinary retention, also occurred. This was associated with paraprostatic cyst prostatitis or malignancy, but prostatic hyperplasia ma also result in incontinence.

The diagnosis and treatment of prostatic disorder are described in Chapter 5.

Bladder/urethral neoplasia

OCCASIONALLY, ANIMALS with bladder neoplasi exhibit urinary incontinence. In the author's experi ence, this has been confined to dogs with carcinomas a various sites in the bladder.

In dogs with bladder neck tumours, urinar retention with overflow incontinence can occur, bu incontinence in these cases can also occur withou retention. It is likely that incontinent dogs with bladde neck/urethral neoplasia have impairment of th sphincter mechanism (**439**), whereas bladder wa tumours (**440**) probably result in detrusor instabilit (see below).

Diagnosis is confirmed by contrast radiograph ultrasonography, cystoscopy and/or cytology/biops but the possibility of malignancy should be eliminate before surgical excision is attempted. Even in th absence of evidence of malignancy, histopathologica examination of the excised tumour is essential to obtai a prognosis.

439 Carcinoma of the bladder neck and proximal urethra (demonstrated by double contrast cystography) of an incontinent dog.

440 Carcinoma of the cranioventral bladder wall (demonstrated by double contrast cystography) of an incontinent dog. Despite the abnormal appearance of the prostatic urethra and prostate gland, there were no abnormalities of these at postmortem examination

Uretero- or vesicovaginal fistula

URETEROVAGINAL FISTULATION IS a complication of spaying in bitches and queens and probably results from inclusion of a ureter during ligation of the cranial vaginal/cervical/uterine stump. An acquired ectopic ureter draining into the vagina results and this can be diagnosed by contrast radiography (**441**). Treatment is identical to that for congenital ureteral ectopia (i.e. ureter transplantation or, if severe secondary ureteral and renal problems are present, ureteronephrectomy), although, sometimes, the adhesed ureter/vagina granuloma can be excised and the ureter ends re-joined (**442–447**).

Rarely, after spaying, vesicovaginal fistulation can occur (**448**). Even rarer, both conditions can occur in the same animal (**449**).

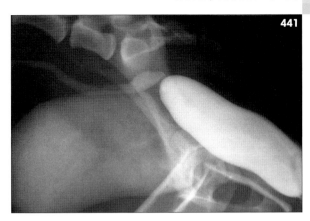

441 Ureterovaginal fistula demonstrated by retrograde positive contrast vagino-urethrography.

442–447 Ureterovaginal fistulectomy and ureteral anastomosis in a juvenile Cocker Spaniel bitch with an iatrogenic ureterovaginal fistula (following ovariohysterectomy).

(**442**) The bladder has been reflected caudally (to the left) and its dorsal wall exposed. The vagina (V) has been elevated and the site of fistulation exposed. Cranial to the granuloma on the anterior vagina, the ureter is identified (arrowed) surrounded by peritoneum and fat. In this animal the insertion of the caudal ureter into the bladder can also be seen (also arrowed); this was not detectable on pre-operative contrast radiography. An intra-operative decision was made to resect the cranial vaginal granuloma and traumatized section of ureter and to perform ureteral anastomosis. If insufficient caudal ureter remains in these cases and/or gross hydroureter (± hydronephrosis) exists, re-implantation of the ureter into the bladder (see **426, 427**) or ureteronephrectomy (see **319–337**) is required.

(**443**) The cranial vagina is ligated and sectioned caudal to the granuloma, as shown.

(**444**) The granuloma containing the ureterovaginal fistula is excised, leaving caudal and cranial sections of ureter, which require anastomosis. Any bleeding ureteral vessels should be clamped and ligated level with the ends of the ureter. The hub of a 3Fr urinary catheter has been cut off and the catheter passed, hub end first, through the caudal ureter (identified by the artery clamps on the ureteral vessel), bladder and urethra to exit at the vulva.

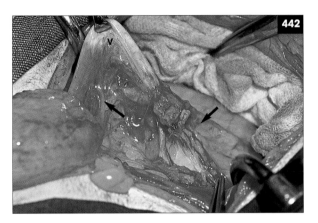

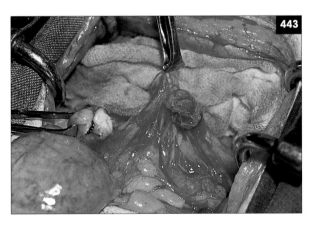

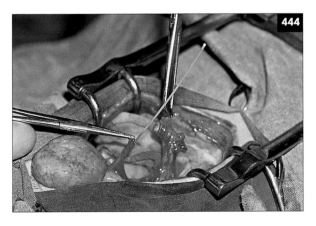

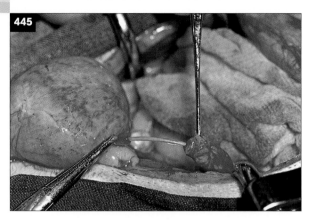

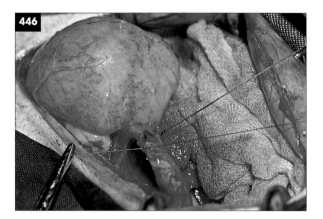

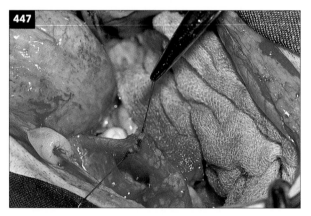

(**445**) The catheter tip is introduced into the cranial section of ureter (being held by fine rat-toothed forceps) and passed cranially to a level just distal to the ureteropelvic junction.

(**446**) The ureter is anastomosed, taking care to avoid rotation of the ureteral sections around their longitudinal axis. Simple interrupted sutures have been placed 180° apart to facilitate orientation and handling. Fine synthetic absorbable sutures (e.g. 5/0 polyglactin) should be used in a simple interrupted pattern. Ureteral surgery is less traumatic and suture placement improved if fine ocular instruments are used.

(**447**) Anastomosis is completed and the ureter observed for leakage during peristalsis. Alternatively, if ureteral peristalsis is poor, a few millilitres of sterile saline can be gently injected up the catheter to test for leaks. Any leakage sites should be sealed by further suturing, as required. Following routine abdominal closure, the catheter is sutured to the paravulval perineal skin, as illustrated in **89**, and left *in situ* for 3–5 days. In some animals, despite being sutured in place, the indwelling ureteral catheter will come out within 72 hours, presumably as a result of ureteral peristalsis and urine flow pressures.

448 Vesicovaginal fistula (arrowed) demonstrated by retrograde positive contrast vagino-urethrography in an incontinent bitch.

449 In this bitch the bladder neck had apparently been included in the vaginal ligature during spaying, resulting in ureterovaginal fistulation and a fistula between the remnants of the bladder (arrowed) and the vagina. The other kidney had ceased to function because of severe hydronephrosis due to the obstruction of the ureter at the trigone. Euthanasia was required in this case.

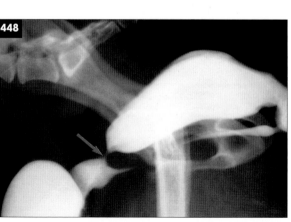

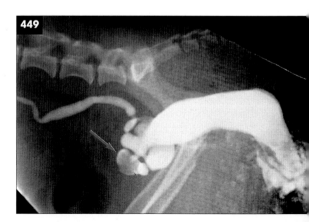

Acquired neurological conditions

AS WITH CONGENITAL neurological conditions, acquired urinary retention with overflow incontinence may result from UMN or LMN dysfunction, usually as a sequela to spinal lesions (e.g. intervertebral disc prolapse, tumours).

Other neurological abnormalities are usually apparent, but if the lesion affects the cauda equina, ambulation may not be grossly affected (see **145–147**). The diagnosis may be confirmed by radiography and advanced imaging techniques such as CT scans or MRI. Treatment is conservative or surgical (spinal) depending on the cause, severity and duration of signs. In the case of tumours, euthanasia is usually performed.

Overflow incontinence with chronic retention

ANIMALS WITH URETHRAL obstruction (e.g. calculi, tumours) may, paradoxically, become incontinent when the intravesical pressure becomes high enough to overcome the urethral resistance. Such cases are primarily presented with dysuria and should be investigated and treated as such (see Chapters 4 and 5).

Detrusor overactivity/hyperactivity/instability

THESE CONDITIONS APPEAR to be very rare in animals. In affected cases, uncontrollable bladder contractions occur, resulting in voiding. Detrusor overactivity is the generic term used for involuntary detrusor contractions, the aetiology of which is unclear. Detrusor hyperactivity (hyperreflexia) denotes involuntary detrusor contractions due to neurological conditions. Detrusor instability is used to describe involuntary detrusor contractions that are not due to neurological causes.

In dogs, detrusor overactivity may be secondary to lesions leading to excessive bladder wall stimulation (e.g. cystitis, bladder tumours). Such stimulation may also occur in animals with bladder hypoplasia, especially if they are housed for long periods and unable to inhibit the detrusor reflex. The owners of such animals may report nocturia or marked bed-wetting overnight.

Detrusor instability can occur with no obvious underlying cause. It may be present alone or in conjunction with urethral sphincter mechanism incompetence. Diagnosis depends upon the taking of a detailed history and elimination of other causes of incontinence. In humans the urodynamic diagnosis of this condition requires considerable patient co-operation and feedback, something that is lacking in veterinary patients!

In cases secondary to other disorders, such as cystitis, treatment of the primary condition alone usually results in a return to continence. Animals with bladder hypoplasia and primary detrusor instability are much more difficult to treat, but anticholinergic (parasympatholytic) or smooth muscle antispasmodic drugs may be beneficial.

Urethral sphincter mechanism incompetence

DURING URINE STORAGE, urethral resistance is maintained by a complex mechanism of factors. These include tone in the urethral smooth muscle (the 'internal' sphincter), tone in the urethral striated muscle (the 'external' sphincter), the natural elasticity of the urethral wall tissues (not only musculature), the physical properties of the urethra (length and diameter) and the degree of engorgement of suburothelial venous plexuses. Since no true bladder neck sphincter exists in the bitch and continence is maintained by a complex mechanism of interacting factors, the term 'urethral sphincter mechanism incompetence' is used to describe a weakness of the urinary sphincter.

The neuromuscular function of the lower urinary tract in the dog is complex and not completely understood. Our current understanding is summarized in **450**.

450 Summary of neuromuscular control of urinary continence. It is likely that most urethral tone is due to the smooth muscle, innervated by the sympathetic nervous system, with the striated muscle being used to augment urethral resistance during times when the intravesical pressure suddenly rises (e.g. during barking). In the cat and human there is also sympathetic innervation to the urethral striated muscle, but this has yet to be demonstrated in the dog. This diagram is an oversimplification of continence control; for example, sympathetic and parasympathetic nerves meet and interact at the same ganglia on the urethral and bladder walls, making understanding of function (to this author at least) difficult.

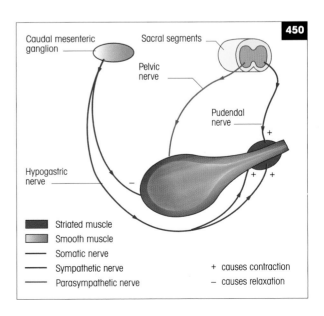

Caudal mesenteric ganglion
Sacral segments
Pelvic nerve
Pudendal nerve
Hypogastric nerve

▮ Striated muscle
▮ Smooth muscle
— Somatic nerve
— Sympathetic nerve
— Parasympathetic nerve

\+ causes contraction
\− causes relaxation

Urethral sphincter mechanism incompetence occurs in dogs and cats, although it is rare in the latter. In dogs referred for investigation of urinary incontinence, urethral sphincter mechanism incompetence is the commonest diagnosis made in adults and is second only to ureteral ectopia in juveniles, particularly in females (**451, 452**).

It can present as a congenital or acquired condition. The acquired form is extremely rare in the cat; in cats most cases of urethral sphincter mechanism incompetence are congenital. Although urethral pressure profilometry can be used to demonstrate incompetence of the urethral sphincter mechanism (see Chapter 3), this technique is not readily available in general practice and is predisposed to a number of artefacts that can make interpretation difficult. In general practice, therefore, the diagnosis is usually made on the basis of the breed and history and by the elimination of other possible diagnoses using imaging and laboratory techniques.

451, 452 Urethral sphincter mechanism incompetence is diagnosed in 80% of dogs referred for the investigation of urinary incontinence (**451**) and is the second commonest cause of congenital urinary incontinence in juvenile dogs (**452**).

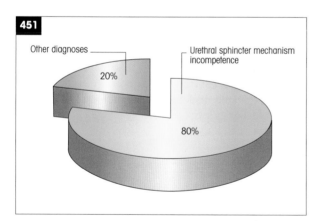

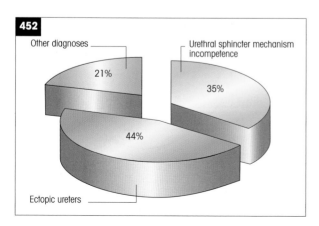

Congenital urethral sphincter mechanism incompetence

IN DOGS, THIS TENDS to be a problem of large breeds, predominantly bitches. Leakage of urine is more copious compared with animals with ureteral ectopia, and it occurs predominantly when the dogs are recumbent (**453**).

The urethra may be abnormally short or even absent, especially in cats (**454–456**), and urethral diverticula and dilatations may be present in juvenile male dogs (**457–461**).

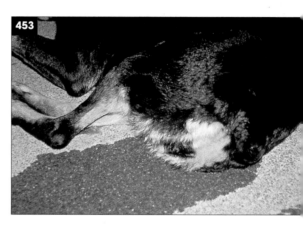

453 Passive leakage of urine during recumbency (in a Rottweiler bitch), typical of urethral sphincter mechanism incompetence.

454–456 Congenital urethral sphincter mechanism incompetence in cats is associated with severe urethral shortening (**454**) or even absence (**455**), with the bladder neck apparently opening directly into the vestibule. Many of these cats have no vagina (**455**); the streak of contrast medium visible dorsal to the bladder neck in this cat represents retrograde filling of the uterine horns, which insert directly into the bladder. A vagino-urethrogram of a normal female cat is shown for comparison (**456**).

457–458 Prostatic urethral diverticulae and a dilated pelvic urethra demonstrated during urethrography (**457**) and at postmortem examination (**458**) in a juvenile Golden Retriever.

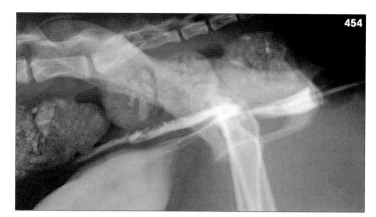

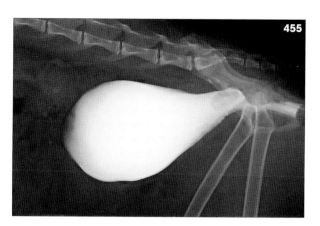

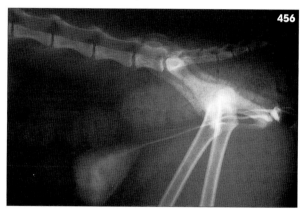

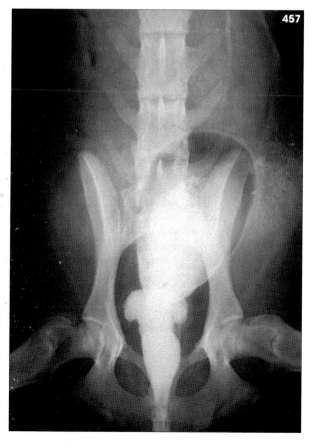

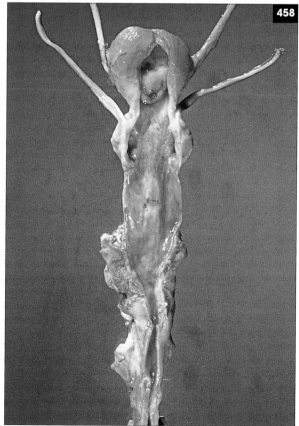

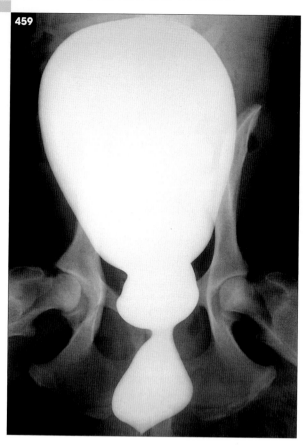

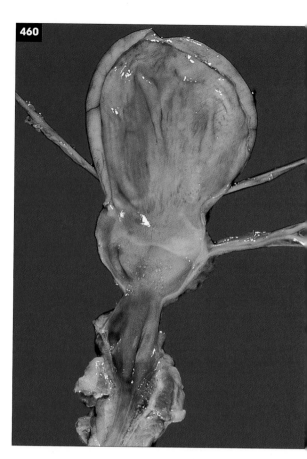

459, 460 Prostatic and pelvic urethral dilatations in an incontinent juvenile German Shepherd Dog demonstrated during urethrography (**459**) and at postmortem examination (**460**).

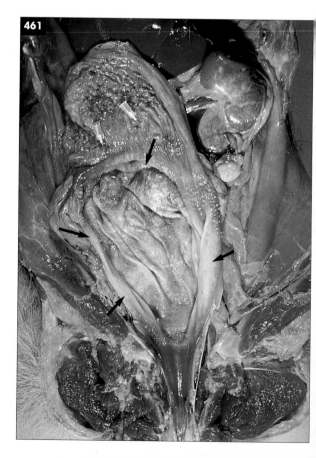

461 The worst case of a prostatic urethral dilatation (arrowed) the author has seen (in a juvenile German Shepherd Dog) demonstrated at postmortem examination.

In many bitches, no gross abnormalities are detected on contrast radiographic investigations, apart from a caudally positioned bladder, and the diagnosis frequently relies on the history and elimination of other possible causes of incontinence. Approximately half of affected bitches become continent following their first or second oestrus and so should not be neutered before then. Those that do not may be candidates for medical or surgical management (see Acquired urethral sphincter mechanism incompetence in bitches). Oestrogens are contraindicated in juvenile bitches with this condition because of possible adverse 'feed-back' effects on the pituitary, but alpha-adrenergics such as phenylpropanolamine could be used, pending oestrus.

In cases of severe urethral hypoplasia, especially in cats, partial bladder neck resection (462–465) or reconstruction may be beneficial. Bladder neck reconstruction is more complicated, but the results are no better than partial bladder neck resection and so the latter is preferred. Approximately half of these cats will be cured by the surgery, although, if the uterine horns insert into the bladder (see 455 and 466), these can cause problems after surgery (467, 468).

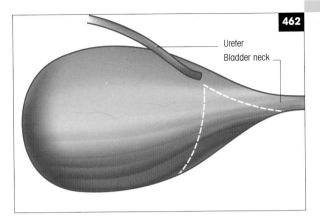

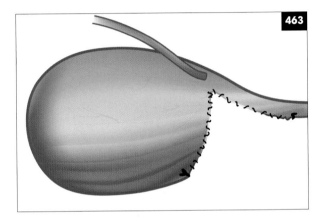

462, 463 Diagrams illustrating bladder neck resection technique. The ventral portion of the bladder neck is excised as far cranially as just distal to the ureteral orifices, to avoid creating an 'ectopic ureter' into the new portion of urethra (**462**). The resulting defect is then repaired to create a longer urethra (**463**).

464, 465 Pre-operative (**464**) and postoperative (**465**) vestibulo-urethrocystography in a cat with urinary incontinence due to severe urethral hypoplasia.

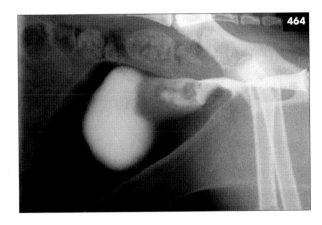

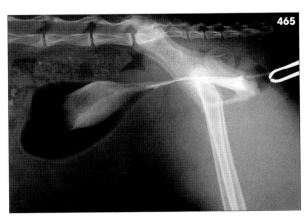

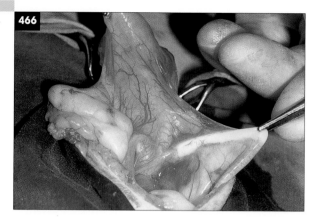

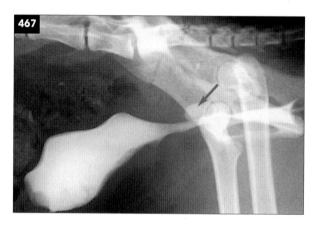

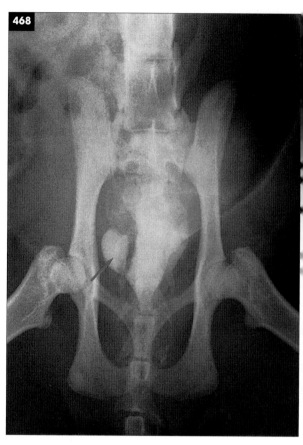

466 In cats with urethral hypoplasia and vaginal aplasia, the uterine horns insert into the bladder at the level of the trigone.

467, 468 Postoperative lateral (**467**) and ventrodorsal (**468**) vestibulo-urethocystograms in a cat with urethral hypoplasia and vaginal aplasia. The uterine horns were excised during surgery, but the uterine horn remnant (arrowed) is acting as a bladder diverticulum, predisposing this cat to recurring urinary tract infections.

Acquired urethral sphincter mechanism incompetence in bitches

ACQUIRED URETHRAL SPHINCTER mechanism incompetence usually (but not always) follows spaying in the bitch and castration in male dogs. Before treatment can be contemplated, an understanding of the pathophysiology of urethral sphincter mechanism incompetence is required. The exact abnormality leading to urethral sphincter mechanism incompetence and the region of the urethra in which it occurs are unknown. It is a multi-factorial problem and a variety of factors are known or suspected to contribute to its clinical manifestation of urinary incontinence. These factors include urethral tone, urethral length, bladder neck position, body size and breed, ovariohysterectomy/ovariectomy, hormones and obesity.

Urethral tone

The introduction of urethral pressure profilometry as an investigative aid in the bitch has allowed confirmation of the belief that poor urethral tone is implicated in urinary incontinence due to urethral sphincter mechanism incompetence. Urethral tone is maintained by a complex interaction of neuromuscular, vascular and passive elastic components, and it is unclear which and/or to what extent each of these is deficient in sphincter mechanism incompetence.

Urethral length

There is considerable variation in urethral length between bitches of different sizes. However, taking body size into consideration, bitches with urethral sphincter mechanism incompetence tend to have shorter urethras than continent animals.

Bladder neck position

A number of authors recorded the radiographic finding of a 'pelvic bladder' during the investigation of incontinent animals (**469, 470**). The significance of this finding was disputed in the past, but there is now good evidence that an intrapelvic bladder neck contributes significantly to urinary incontinence due to urethral sphincter mechanism incompetence. The caudal bladder position in affected dogs is associated with the shorter urethral length and also the fact that the bladder moves caudally when a bitch moves from a standing to a relaxed recumbent position. This movement is more pronounced in bitches with urethral sphincter mechanism incompetence than in normal animals, suggesting a deficiency in supporting mechanisms in the lower urinary tract of affected animals. The role of bladder neck position in bitches with urethral sphincter mechanism incompetence is thought to be due to changes in transference of abdominal pressures to the urethra (**471, 472**).

469, 470 (**469**) The so-called 'pelvic bladder' demonstrated by retrograde positive contrast vagino-urethrography in an adult, spayed Rough Collie with urethral sphincter mechanism incompetence (this bitch also has a vestibulovaginal stricture).
(**470**) A vagino-urethrogram of an adult, spayed, continent Rough Collie is provided for comparison.

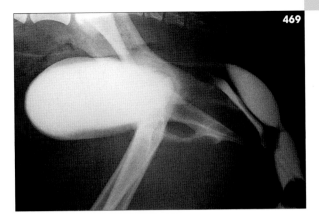

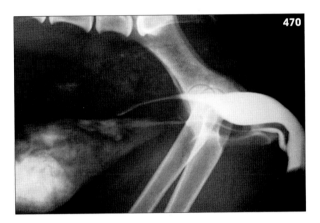

471, 472 In a bitch with an intra-abdominal bladder neck (**471**), any pressure changes in the abdomen (grey arrows) are transmitted to both the bladder and the urethra (brown arrows), so tending to cancel each other out. Such an animal may be able to cope better with an incompetent urethral sphincter mechanism. In most bitches with an incompetent bladder sphincter, the bladder neck is intrapelvic (**472**) and so intra-abdominal pressures are transmitted more to the bladder than the urethra, creating a pressure gradient. If the urethral sphincter mechanism is incompetent, this can result in urine leakage when intra-abdominal pressure rises, for example during recumbency.

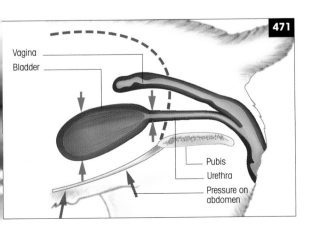

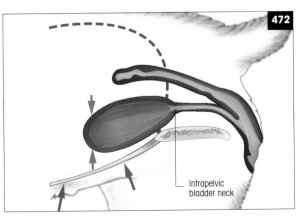

Body size and breed

LARGE AND GIANT BREEDS are at risk. Urethral sphincter mechanism incompetence is commonest in the UK in Dobermanns and Old English Sheepdogs, and there is evidence that these breeds and also Rottweilers, Weimaraners, Springer Spaniels and Irish Setters, are particularly at risk.

Ovariohysterectomy/ovariectomy and hormones

THERE IS AN ASSOCIATION between spaying and urinary incontinence and this is probably due to a lack of circulating oestrogens, although a recent paper suggests that an excess of gonadotrophins may also be a factor. In general terms, spayed animals are nearly eight times more likely to develop this form of urinary incontinence than entire bitches. However, this should be considered in terms of dog years. In simple terms, if 100 bitches were not spayed, ten years later, two of them would be incontinent. If 100 bitches were spayed, about 16 of them would be incontinent after ten years. Spaying before the first season may increase the risk, although this could not be proved conclusively in a prospective study, probably because of the low number of animals examined. A recent paper suggested that if early gonadectomy of female dogs is practised, it should be delayed until the animal is at least three months of age. The function and morphometry of the lower urinary tract are affected by the changes in hormone balance that occur during the oestrus cycle.

Obesity

WHILST NOT A CAUSE of the condition, obesity may worsen the degree of incontinence and weight loss may improve the situation.

Vestibulovaginal stenosis in relation to urethral sphincter mechanism incompetence in bitches

VESTIBULOVAGINAL STENOSIS, due to a true stricture (see **469**) or persistent perforate hymen, has been linked to urinary incontinence by some authors. It was initially suggested that the incontinence might be associated with urine accumulating cranial to the stenosis during micturition and subsequently dribbling out. However, research later revealed no difference in the prevalence of vestibulovaginal stenosis between normal an incontinent bitches, and the author now believes tha vestibulovaginal stenosis *per se* is not a cause of incont nence, although if a bitch is already incontinent an leaking urine into the vagina, some may accumulat cranial to the stenosis, exacerbating the signs and pre disposing to vaginitis. Experience suggests that th incontinence is due to other causes such as urethra sphincter mechanism incompetence and that if th incontinence due to these can be cured, the vestibulo vaginal stenosis is irrelevant.

Urethral sphincter mechanism incompetence in male dogs

URETHRAL SPHINCTER mechanism incompetence i male dogs is uncommon. As in the bitch, the conditio can occur as either a congenital or an acquired condition. The congenital condition is often associated with gross prostatic/pelvic urethral deformities (urethra dilatations and prostatic urethral diverticulae) and i unlikely to be successfully treated (see **457–461**). Again as in the bitch, the acquired form is associated with neutering and larger breeds appear to be at risk. Incontinence is likely to occur when intra-abdomina pressure increases (e.g. during recumbency) and affected animals tend to have intrapelvic bladder necks, although a short urethra does not appear to be a factor in males. Conservative management is frequently disappointing. In comparison with the bitch, the condition is less likely to respond to medical therapy. The pathophysiology o male urethral sphincter mechanism incompetence is poorly understood, making rational treatment difficult. Drugs used in its management include androgens, oestrogens and alpha-adrenergics. Of these, alpha-adrenergics ± estrogens give the best results, but, even then, more than half of the dogs fail to respond to therapy. Attempts have been made to relocate the intrapelvic bladder neck to an intra-abdominal position. These have involved pexy of the deferent ducts to the abdominal wall or prostatopexy (in castrated males) to the prepubic tendon. As with medical treatment, the impression in a limited number of cases is that surgical treatment alone of urethral sphincter mechanism incompetence is less successful in males than in bitches.

Treatment of urethral sphincter mechanism incompetence

THE TREATMENT OF congenital urethral sphincter mechanism incompetence has been mentioned previously. Since it is a multifactorial problem, the treatment of acquired urethral sphincter mechanism incompetence may be difficult and most therapies correct only one of the factors described previously. It is unlikely, therefore, that any one form of treatment alone will cure 100% of cases in the long term. A good figure to bear in mind is 50%. A close look at the literature suggests this is the cure rate that can be expected for any one form of treatment of this condition, be it medical or surgical, although most of the remaining animals are improved by treatment.

In theory, sympathomimetic or parasympatholytic agents should improve continence control by increasing urethral tone or reducing intravesical pressure respectively (see **450**). Oestrogens have also been used to improve urethral tone. Most published clinical trials have involved the efficacy of alpha-adrenergics or oestrogens and tend to have short follow-up periods. In addition, possible long-term adverse systemic effects have not been evaluated. Currently, the most popular medical treatments are the alpha-adrenergic phenyl-propanolamine or oestrogens such as oestriol. In some animals that respond initially to alpha-adrenergics or oestrogens, the response ceases eventually, in the case of oestrogens possibly due to desensitization of oestrogen receptors. Oestrogens sensitize the urethral smooth muscle to alpha-adrenergic stimulation and so a combination of oestrogen and alpha-adrenergic therapy may be useful in animals that have failed to respond to an individual drug and may reduce the dose of each individual drug, lessening the chances of side-effects. Androgens have been employed in castrated male dogs but, in the author's experience, the results are disappointing.

The main options for surgical treatment are to attempt to:

- Increase urethral resistance (e.g. peri-urethral surgical slings or artificial sphincters; intra-urethral injection of bulking agents [**473**]).
- Increase urethral length, using bladder neck reconstruction techniques; this is more commonly used in cats with severe urethral hypoplasia than in dogs (see **462–465**).
- Relocate the bladder neck to an intra-abdominal position by means of colposuspension (**474–484**), urethropexy (**485**), vas deferentopexy or prostatopexy (**486–489**).

The author's preferred technique in bitches is colposuspension, and this will be described in more detail (**474–484**).

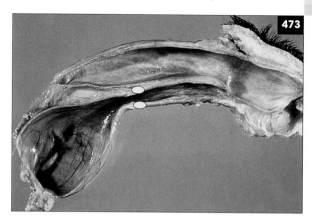

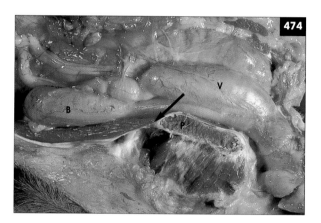

473 Urethral resistance can be increased by injection of urethral bulking agents (polytetrafluoroethylene or collagen) – indicated above by yellow ellipses – into the urethral wall. Polytetrafluoroethylene has been associated with formation of distant granulomas in humans and so collagen is preferable. This technique requires specialized (urethrocystoscopic) equipment.

474 During colposuspension, the vagina (V) on either side of the urethra is anchored to the prepubic tendon in order to move the lower urogenital tract in a cranial direction and relocate the bladder neck in an intra-abdominal position; this improves the transference of abdominal pressures to the bladder neck and proximal urethra (see **471, 472**).
B = bladder; P = pubis.

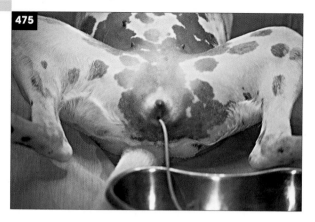

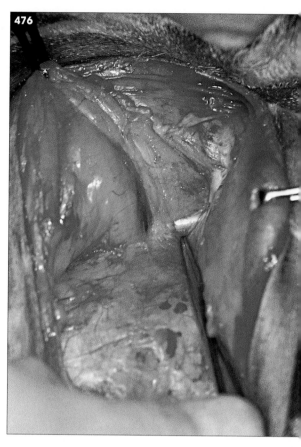

475–484 Colposuspension technique. (**475**) Under general anaesthesia, the bitch is placed in dorsal recumbency with the hindlimbs flexed. The ventral abdominal skin and vagina have been prepared for aseptic surgery, the vagina by douching with dilute aqueous povidone iodine. An 8Fr (smaller bitches) or 10Fr (larger bitches) Foley catheter is inserted via the urethra into the bladder and the cuff inflated. The catheter is then gently withdrawn until the cuff rests in the bladder neck. The presence of the catheter facilitates identification of the urethra and bladder neck during surgery.

(**476**) A midline, caudal abdominal approach is made. The prepubic fat and fascia are separated by careful blunt and sharp dissection on both sides of the midline and the prepubic tendons and external pudendal vessels identified. In the photograph, the bitch's vulva is in the top right corner and the artery forceps point to the left prepubic tendon. Just lateral to the prepubic tendon, the external pudendal vessels can be seen on the edge of the prepubic fat. These vessels must be identified and avoided during subsequent placement of sutures around the prepubic tendon.

(**477**) The midline incision is continued through the linea alba of the abdominal muscle wall and extended caudally to the pubic brim. Self-retaining retractors are used to separate the abdominal musculature and the bladder is identified.

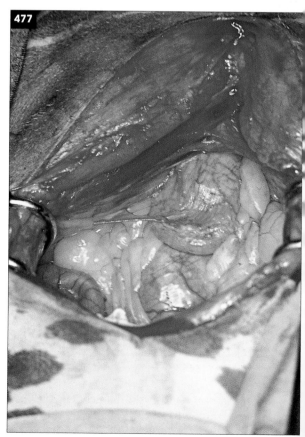

478) Cranial traction on the bladder allows the [in]trapelvic bladder neck (N) to be pulled cranially and [id]entified by the presence of the inflated Foley [ca]theter cuff. Note the presence of the retroperitoneal [fat] around the bladder neck and urethra.

479) The vagina is displaced cranially and cleared of [fat] and fascia on either side of the urethra. Vaginal [di]splacement is most easily accomplished by inserting [a] finger into the vagina. The urethra can be palpated [th]rough the ventral vaginal wall and displaced to the [bi]tch's left, while the vaginal wall (V) over the finger [up] to the right of the urethra is pushed cranially and [ve]ntrally towards the caudal end of the incision. The [va]ginal wall can then be exposed by pushing off the [o]verlying fat and fascia in a caudal direction using a [dr]y swab. The bladder neck (N) can be seen as a [s]welling due to the presence of the Foley catheter cuff [in] the bladder. The vaginal wall is grasped with tissue [fo]rceps. The technique is repeated on the other side of [th]e urethra. The surgeon then changes his/her gloves [an]d the vulva is covered with a large sterile swab or [su]rgical drape throughout the remainder of the [p]rocedure. In bitches in which one's finger and the [v]agina are of incompatible sizes (very large or very [sm]all bitches or those with gross vaginal strictures or [se]ptae), the vagina has to be located by blunt and [s]harp dissection of the overlying fat and fascia on [ei]ther side of the urethra, grasped with tissue forceps [a]nd then pulled cranially. Placement of a long, thin [bl]unt instrument (e.g. a Poole suction tip) into the [v]agina facilitates identification. This is more difficult [th]an the use of a finger in the vagina and, fortunately, [m]ost bitches with urethral sphincter mechanism [in]competence are of a size that is usually compatible [w]ith one's finger, depending on the size of the finger, [o]f course.

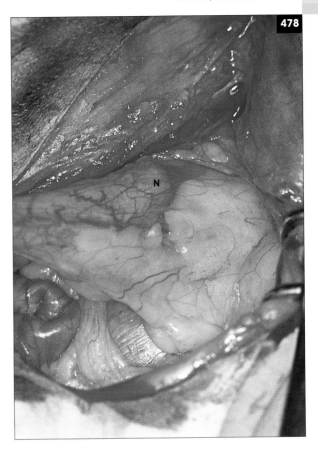

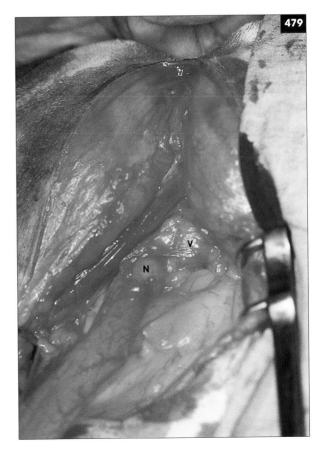

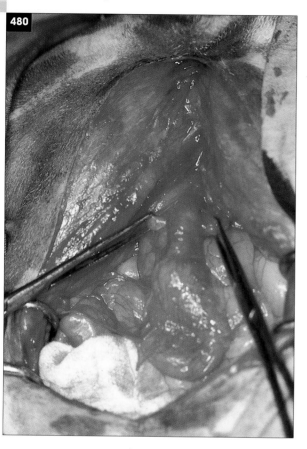

(**480**) In this illustration the vagina on either side of the urethra has been grasped with Allis tissue forceps and pulled cranially. As can be seen, this results in movement of the bladder neck and proximal urethra from an intrapelvic to an intra-abdominal position. (The swab in the abdomen is not essential and was used to prevent small intestine from obscuring part o: the photographic field).

(**481**) If the tension on the tissue forceps is released, the cranial vagina and bladder neck move back to an intrapelvic position. The vagina must therefore be anchored cranially to maintain the bladder neck in an intra-abdominal position.

(**482**) The vagina is sutured to the prepubic tendon o: each side of and approximately 1–1.5 cm away from the midline. The sutures (monofilament nylon) are taken through the abdominal wall caudal to the tendon, in and out of the vaginal wall (as far laterally as possible) and back out of the abdominal wall crania: to the tendon. The placement of a suture attaching the left vaginal wall to the left prepubic tendon is illustrated. It is possible that the sutures may enter the vaginal lumen during this procedure, hence the need for preparation of the vagina for aseptic surgery.

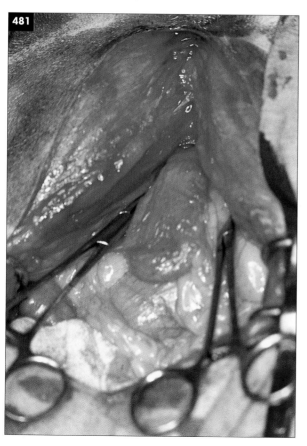

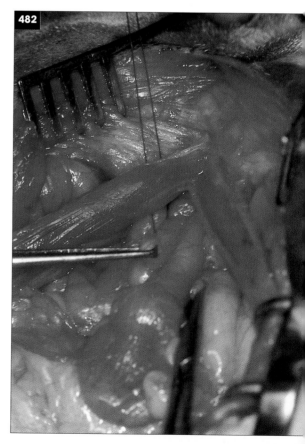

(**483**) The number of sutures that can be placed around the prepubic tendon depends on the size of the bitch and is limited by the external pudendal vessels laterally. Most bitches are medium to large breeds and the optimum number of sutures is two on each side, as illustrated. No. 0 nylon is suitable for most bitches but no. 1 nylon should be used in very large breeds. On the rare occasions when colposuspension is performed in small or toy breeds, it may only be possible to place one suture through the vagina and around the prepubic tendon on either side of the mid-line. Once the sutures have been placed, they are pulled tight to ensure that after they are tied, the urethra will not be compressed against the pubis by an arch of vagina, since this may result in postoperative dysuria. It should be possible to insert the tip of a blunt-ended instrument, such as Mayo scissors or Kilner needle holders, easily alongside the urethra between the vaginal arch and pubis. If the urethra is compressed, the sutures should be repositioned, but this is not usually necessary if the sutures have been placed as laterally on the vagina as possible. If all is well, the sutures are tied, the Foley catheter removed and the abdomen closed routinely.

(**484**) The vagina will form adhesions to the abdominal wall near the prepubic tendon. This is the postmortem appearance of a bitch eight years after a colposuspension. A metal probe has been inserted into the urethra and used to elevate it, better to demonstrate the vaginal adhesion (arrowed).
V = vagina; B = bladder; P = pubis.

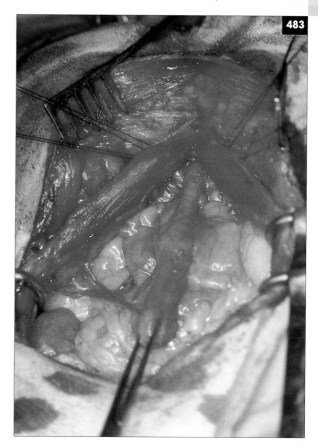

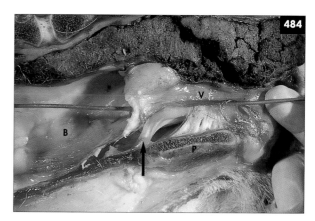

485 During urethropexy, the urethra is anchored to the prepubic tendon or abdominal muscle wall (arrowed).
V = vagina; B = bladder; P = pubis.

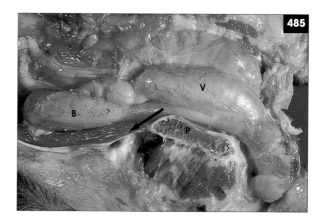

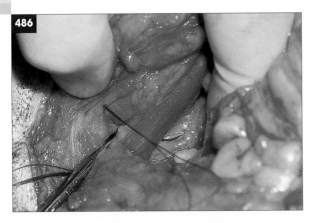

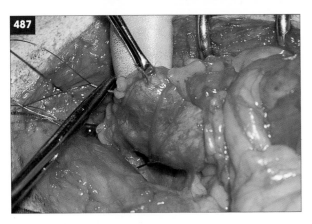

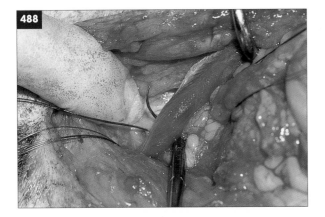

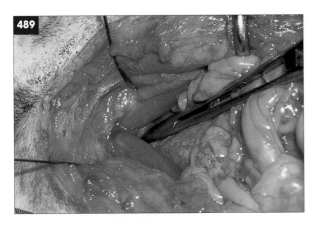

486–489 Prostatopexy is the male equivalent of colposuspension, except that the prostate is anchored to the prepubic tendon on either side of the urethra rather than the vagina. After the suture has been introduced through the abdominal wall caudal to the prepubic tendon (**486**), a bite is taken through the caudoventral edge of the prostate gland on the same side (**487**). The same suture is then taken back out though the abdominal wall, cranial to the prepubic tendon (**488**). This is repeated on the opposite side with two sutures being placed on each side and assessed to ensure there is no urethral compression, as in colposuspension (**489**).

The potential problem with techniques intended to increase urethral resistance is that they may increase morbidity by making an incontinent animal dysuric. Similarly, increasing urethral length carries potentially serious surgical risks and, in the author's view, should be reserved for animals with severe congenital urethral hypoplasia. The technique least likely to lead to serious complications is to relocate the bladder neck to an intra-abdominal position by means of colposuspension. The greater experience of medical urologists treating incontinent women suggests that colposuspension provides firmer anchorage of the lower urogenital tract than urethropexy and avoids urethral trauma. It may also prevent the caudal movement of the bladder that occurs during recumbency and is more pronounced in bitches with urethral sphincter mechanism incompetence. However, a review of urethropexy as a treatment for urethral sphincter mechanism incompetence in 100 bitches revealed similar results to colposuspension, although the prevalence and severity of urethral complications was higher. The author believes that cystopexy is contraindicated in these cases, since it may result in detrusor instability, a further cause of urinary incontinence.

The complications after colposuspension are few and most are relatively minor. Since the surgery involves trauma to intrapelvic structures, some animals are stimulated to strain, usually immediately after recovery from the general anaesthetic. This can be controlled by the administration of appropriate analgesics pre-, peri- and postoperatively. Rarely, some bitches find the first defaecation after surgery to be uncomfortable if the faeces are firm and bulky. This can be controlled with stool softeners. The commonest complication is dysuria, but this occurs in less than 3% of cases in the author's experience. It may be due to vaginal stimulation by the surgery leading to suppression of the micturition reflex and/or reflex dyssynergia.

Clinical observations and the response to diazepam suggest that reflex voluntary dyssynergia is the most likely cause of dysuria after colposuspension. It may be exacerbated by recent oestrogen therapy and so any oestrogen therapy should cease at least one month pre-operatively. Voluntary dyssynergia usually responds to diazepam at a dose of 0.2 mk/kg by mouth two or three times daily. The drug has a short duration of action and so each dose should be given 15–20 minutes before the animal is walked to urinate. An indwelling urinary catheter can be used for a few days, if necessary, in the minority of animals that are unable to urinate at all. A further potential cause of dysuria is compression of the urethra against the pubis by the vagina. Care should be taken during surgery to avoid placement of vaginal sutures too close to the urethra (see **483**). Bitches that are allowed to be very active after colposuspension may tear the sutures from the vagina. This is more likely to happen if they are allowed to run and jump, and owners should be advised of the necessity for restricting the exercise of their animals to walks on the lead only for one month after surgery. Hymen formation and accumulation of vaginal secretions causing dysuria and/or dyschezia is an extremely rare, longer-term complication of colposuspension. It is due to breakdown of a pre-existing vestibulo-vaginal stricture during the operation and subsequent healing of apposing raw areas of vagina to form a barrier across the vaginal lumen.

Although great progress has been made over the past three decades in our understanding of the pathophysiology and, thus, the treatment of canine urethral sphincter mechanism incompetence, a recent editorial by one of the world's most respected urologists suggests we still have a great deal to learn. Despite over 200 procedures being described for the treatment of human stress incontinence, the author was left asking, when it comes to his own patients, what should he do?

References and further reading

Part 1: Investigation of animals with urological signs

Atalan G, Barr FJ, Holt PE (1998) Assessment of bladder volume in dogs by use of linear ultrasonographic measurements. *American Journal of Veterinary Research* **59**, 10–15.

Atalan G, Barr FJ, Holt PE (1998) Assessment of bladder volume using ultrasonographic determination of cross-sectional areas and linear measurements. *Veterinary Radiology & Ultrasound* **39**, 446–450.

Atalan G, Holt PE, Barr FJ (1999) Effect of body position on ultrasonographic estimations of bladder volume. *Journal of Small Animal Practice* **40**, 177–179.

Atalan G, Holt PE, Barr FJ (1999) Ultrasonographic estimation of prostate size in normal dogs and relationship to bodyweight and age. *Journal of Small Animal Practice* **40**, 119–122.

Atalan G, Barr FJ, Holt PE (1999) Comparison of ultrasonographic and radiographic measurements of canine prostate dimensions. *Veterinary Radiology & Ultrasound* **40**, 408–412.

Barr FJ, Holt PE, Gibbs C (1990) Ultrasonographic measurement of normal renal parameters. *Journal of Small Animal Practice* **31**, 180–184.

Barthez PY, Smeak DD, Wisner ER *et al.* (2000) Ureteral obstruction after ureteroneocystostomy in dogs assessed by Technetium Tc 99m diethylenetriamine pantaacetic acid (DTPA) scintigraphy. *Veterinary Surgery* **29**, 499–506.

Billett JP, Hotson Moore A, Holt PE (2002) Evaluation of a bladder tumour antigen test for the diagnosis of lower urinary tract malignancies in dogs. *American Journal of Veterinary Research* **63**, 370–373.

Brearley MJ, Cooper JE, Sullivan M (1991) *A Colour Atlas of Small Animal Endoscopy*. Wolfe Publishing, London, pp. 77–86.

Cannizzo KL, McLoughlin MA, Mattoon JS *et al.* (2003) Evaluation of transurethral cystoscopy and excretory urography for diagnosis of ectopic ureters in female dogs: 25 cases (1992–2000). *Journal of the American Veterinary Medical Association* **223**, 475–481.

Gatoria IS, Saini NS, Rai TS *et al.* (2006) Comparison of three techniques for the diagnosis of urinary tract infections in dogs with urolithiasis. *Journal of Small Animal Practice* **47**, 727–732.

Gregory SP, Holt PE, Parkinson TJ (1992) Comparison of two catheter withdrawal speeds during simultaneous urethral pressure profilometry in anesthetized bitches. *American Journal of Veterinary Research* **53**, 355–358.

Gregory SP, Cripps PJ, Holt PE (1996) Comparison of urethral pressure profilometry and contrast radiography in the diagnosis of incompetence of the urethral sphincter mechanism in bitches. *Veterinary Record* **138**, 58–61.

Grooters AM, Cuypers M-LD, Partington BP *et al.* (1997) Renomegally in dogs and cats. Part II. Diagnostic approach. *Compendium on Continuing Education for the Practising Veterinarian* **19**, 1213–1229.

Hamaide AJ, Verstegen JP, Snaps FR *et al.* (2003) Validation and comparison of the use of diuresis cystometry and retrograde filling cystometry at various infusion rates in female Beagle dogs. *American Journal of Veterinary Research* **64**, 574–579.

Henry CJ, Tyler JW, McEntee MC *et al.* (2003) Antigen testing for transitional cell carcinoma in dogs. *American Journal of Veterinary Research* **64**, 1017–1020.

Holt PE (1989) Positive contrast vagino-urethrography for diagnosis of lower urinary tract disease. In *Current Veterinary Therapy X. Small Animal Practice.* (ed RW Kirk) WB Saunders, Philadelphia, pp. 1142–1145.

Holt PE (1990) Simultaneous urethral pressure profilometry using microtip transducer catheters in the bitch: a comparison of catheter materials. *Journal of Small Animal Practice* **31**, 431–436.

Holt PE, Gibbs C, Latham J (1984) An evaluation of positive contrast vagino-urethrography as a diagnostic aid in the bitch. *Journal of Small Animal Practice* **25**, 531–549.

Holt PE, Gibbs C, Wathes CM (1990) Simultaneous urethral pressure profilometry using a microtip transducer catheter in the bitch: effects of bitch position and transducer orientation. *Neurourology and Urodynamics* **9**, 281–296.

Holt PE, Gregory SP (1993) Resting urethral pressure profilometry in bitches: artefact or reality? *Compendium on Continuing Education for the Practising Veterinarian* **15**, 1207–1215.

Mannion P (2006) (ed) *Diagnostic Ultrasound in Small Animal Practice*. Blackwell Publishing, Oxford.

McCarthy TC (2005) Cystoscopy. In *Veterinary Endoscopy for the Small Animal Practitioner*. (ed TC McCarthy) Elsevier Science, St. Louis, pp. 49–135.

Melhoff T, Osborne CA (1977) Catheter biopsy of the urethra, urinary bladder and prostate gland. In *Current Veterinary Therapy VI. Small Animal Practice*. (ed RW Kirk) WB Saunders, Philadelphia, pp. 1173–1175.

Rivers BJ, Walter PA, Polzin DJ (1997) Ultrasonographic-guided, percutaneous antegrade pyelography: technique and clinical application in the dog and cat. *Journal of the American Animal Hospital Association* **33**, 61–68.

Rozear L, Tidwell AS (2003) Evaluation of the ureter and ureterovesicular junction using helical computed tomographic excretory urography in healthy dogs. *Veterinary Radiology & Ultrasound* **44**, 155–164.

Senior DF (1999) Cystoscopy. In *Small Animal Endoscopy*. (ed TR Tams) Mosby, St. Louis, pp. 447–459.

Vaden SL, Levine JF, Lees GE *et al.* (2005) Renal biopsy: a retrospective study of methods and complications in 283 dogs and 65 cats. *Journal of Veterinary Internal Medicine* **19**, 794–801.

Vonderen IK van, Kooistra HS, Rijnberk A (1997) Intra- and interindividual variations in urine osmolality and urine specific gravity in healthy pet dogs of various ages. *Journal of Veterinary Internal Medicine* **11**, 30–35.

Weaver AD (1977) Transperineal punch biopsy of the canine prostate gland. *Journal of Small Animal Practice* **18**, 573–577.

Welles EG, Whatley EM, Hall AS *et al.* (2005) Comparison of Multistix PRO dipsticks with other biochemical assays for determining urine protein (UP), urine creatinine (UC) and UP:UC ratio in dogs and cats. *Veterinary Clinical Pathology* **35**, 31–36.

Part 2: Differential diagnosis and treatment

Chapter 4: Non-prostatic dysuria

Albasan H, Lulich JP, Osborne CA *et al.* (2005) Evaluation of the association between sex and risk of forming urate uroliths in Dalmatians. *Journal of the American Veterinary Medical Association* **227**, 565–569.

Atalan G, Barr FJ, Holt PE (1999) Frequency of urination and ultrasonographic estimation of residual urine in normal and dysuric dogs. *Research in Veterinary Science* **68**, 295–299.

Bass M, Howard J, Gerber B *et al.* (2005) Retrospective study of indications for and outcome of perineal urethrostomy in cats. *Journal of Small Animal Practice* **46**, 227–231.

Bernarde A, Viguier E (2004) Transpelvic urethrostomy in 11 cats using an ischial ostectomy. *Veterinary Surgery* **33**, 246–252.

Bradshaw JM, Brown PJ, Pearson GR *et al.* (1996) Dysuria associated with urethral caruncle in the dog. *Journal of Comparative Pathology* **115**, 77–84.

Davidson EB, Ritchey JW, Higbee RD *et al.* (2004) Laser lithotripsy for treatment of canine uroliths. *Veterinary Surgery* **33**, 56–61.

Davis GJ, Holt D (2003) Two chondrosarcomas in the urethra of a German Shepherd Dog. *Journal of Small Animal Practice* **44**, 169–171.

Diaz Espineira MM, Viehoff FW, Nickel RF (1998) Idiopathic detrusor-urethral dyssynergia in dogs: a retrospective analysis of 22 cases. *Journal of Small Animal Practice* **39**, 264–270.

Dudley RM, Wilkens BE (2004) Urethral obstruction as a complication of staged bilateral triple pelvic osteotomy. *Journal of the American Animal Hospital Association* **40**, 162–164.

Elwick KE, Melendez LD, Higbee RG *et al.* (2003) Neodmium: Yttrium-Aluminum-Garnet (Nd:YAG) laser ablation of an obstructive urethral polyp in a dog. *Journal of the American Animal Hospital Association* **39**, 506–508.

Finkbeiner A, Lapides J (1974) Effect of distension on blood flow in dog's urinary bladder. *Investigative Urology* **12**, 210–212.

Fischer JR, Lane IF, Cribb AE (2003) Urethral pressure profile and haemodynamic effects of phenoxybenzamine and prazosin in non-sedated male Beagle dogs. *Canadian Journal of Veterinary Research* **67**, 30–38.

Gerber B, Boretti FS, Kley S *et al.* (2005) Evaluation of clinical signs and causes of lower urinary tract disease in European cats. *Journal of Small Animal Practice* **46**, 571–577.

Greenberg CB, Davidson EB, Bellmer DD *et al.* (2004) Evaluation of the tensile strengths of four monofilament absorbable suture materials after immersion in canine urine with or without bacteria. *American Journal of Veterinary Research* **65**, 847–853.

Gunn-Moore D (2001) Pathophysiology of feline lower urinary tract disease (FLUTD). *UK Vet* **6**(5), 20–32.

Gunn-Moore D, Brown PJ, Holt PE *et al.* (1995) Priapism in seven cats. *Journal of Small Animal Practice* **36**, 262–266.

Haugaard N, Wein AJ, Chandy B *et al.* (1996) Properties of Ca^{2+}-Mg^{2+} ATP-ase in rabbit bladder muscle and mucosa: effect of urinary outlet obstruction. *Neurourology and Urodynamics* **15**, 555–561.

Hayashi, K, Hardie RJ (2003) Use of cystostomy tubes in small animals. *Compendium on Continuing Education for the Practising Veterinarian* **25**, 928–934.

Hypolite JA, Longhurst PA, Haugaard N *et al.* (1997) Effect of partial outlet obstruction on ^{14}C-adenine incorporation in the rabbit urinary bladder. *Neurourology and Urodynamics* **16**, 201–208.

Kato K, Lin AT-L, Haugaard N *et al.* (1990) Effects of outlet obstruction on glucose metabolism of the rabbit urinary bladder. *Journal of Urology* **143**, 844–847.

Kim JC, Yoon JY, Seo S II *et al.* (2000) Effects of partial bladder outlet obstruction and its relief on types I and III collagen and detrusor contractility in the rat. *Neurourology and Urodynamics* **19**, 29–42.

Lane IF, Fischer JR, Miller E *et al.* (2000) Functional urethral obstruction in 3 dogs: clinical and urethral pressure profile findings. *Journal of Veterinary Internal Medicine* **14**, 43–49.

Lekcharoensuk C, Osborne CA, Lulich JP *et al.* (2002) Associations between dietary factors in canned food and formation of calcium oxalate uroliths in dogs. *American Journal of Veterinary Research* **63**, 163–169.

Levin RM, Malkowicz SB, Wein AJ *et al.* (1985) Recovery from short-term obstruction of the rabbit urinary bladder. *Journal of Urology* **134**, 388–390.

Levin RM, Hypolite JA, Haugaard N *et al.* (1996) Comparative response of rabbit bladder smooth muscle and mucosa to anoxia. *Neurourology and Urodynamics* **15**, 79–84.

Lin AD-Y, Levin R, Kogan B *et al.* (2006) Estrogen induced functional hypertrophy and increased force generation of the female rabbit bladder. *Neurourology and Urodynamics* **25**, 473–479.

Lin AT-L, Yang CH, Chen K-K *et al.* (2005) Detrusor mitochondrial lipid peroxidation and superoxide dismutase activity in partial bladder outlet obstruction of rabbits. *Neurourology and Urodynamics* **24**, 282–287.

Lipscomb V (2004) Surgery of the lower urinary tract in dogs: 2. Urethral surgery. *In Practice* **26**, 13–19.

Lulich JP, Osborne CA, Thumchai R *et al.* (1998) Management of canine calcium oxalate urolith recurrence. *Compendium on Continuing Education for the Practising Veterinarian* **20**, 178–189.

Mannikarottu A, Lin AD-Y, Whitebeck C *et al.* (2006) Effect of partial bladder outlet obstruction on nitrotyrosine levels and their correlation with contractile function. *Neurourology and Urodynamics* **25**, 397–401.

Papadopoulos G, Tommasini Degna M (2006) Two cases of dysuria as a complication of single-session bilateral triple pelvic osteotomy. *Journal of Small Animal Practice* **47**, 741–743.

Pavletic MM, O'Bell SA (2007) Subtotal penile amputation and preputial urethrostomy in a dog. *Journal of the American Veterinary Medical Association* **230**, 375–377.

Piermattei DL, Osborne CA (1977) Urohydropropulsion: non-surgical removal of urethral calculi in male dogs. In *Current Veterinary Therapy VI. Small Animal Practice.* (ed RW Kirk) WB Saunders, Philadelphia, pp. 1194–1196.

Saito M, Ohmura M, Kondo A (1996) Effects of long-term partial outflow obstruction on bladder function in the rat. *Neurourology and Urodynamics* **15**, 157–165.

Salinardi BJ, Marjs SL, Davidson JR *et al.* (2003) The use of a low–profile cystostomy tube to relieve urethral obstruction in a dog. *Journal of the American Animal Hospital Association* **39**, 403–405.

Seaman R, Bartges JW (2001) Canine struvite urolithiasis. *Compendium on Continuing Education for the Practising Veterinarian* **23**, 407–420.

Simpkin P (2005) The Dalmatian defect. *Arthritis and Rheumatism* **52**, 2257–2262.

Stiffler KS, McCrackin Stevenson MA, Sanchez S *et al.* (2006) Prevalence and characterization of urinary tract infections in dogs with surgically treated type I thoracolumbar intervertebral disc extrusion. *Veterinary Surgery* **35**, 330–336.

Takagi S, Kadosawa T, Ishiguro T *et al.* (2005) Urethral transitional cell carcinoma in a cat. *Journal of Small Animal Practice* **46**, 504–506.

Williams JM, White RAS (1991) Tube cystostomy in the dog and cat. *Journal of Small Animal Practice* **32**, 598–602.

Wolffenbuttel KP, Kok DJ, Minekus JPJ *et al.* (2001) Urodynamic follow-up of experimental urethral obstruction in individual guinea pigs. *Neurourology and Urodynamics* **20**, 699–713.

Chapter 5: Prostatic disorders

Boland LE, Hardie RJ, Gregory SP *et al.* (2003) Ultrasound-guided percutaneous drainage as the primary treatment for prostatic abscesses and cysts in dogs. *Journal of the American Animal Hospital Association* **39**, 151–159.

Bommer N (2006) A review of the pathophysiology of prostatic diseases. *UK Vet* **11(3)**, 20–26.

Bommer N (2006) Treatment of prostatic diseases. *UK Vet* **11(4)**, 17–23.

Bray JP, White RAS, Williams JM (1997) Partial resection and omentalisation: a new technique for management of prostatic retention cysts in dogs. *Veterinary Surgery* **26**, 202–209.

Caney SMA, Holt PE, Day MJ *et al.* (1998) Prostatic carcinoma in two cats. *Journal of Small Animal Practice* **39**, 140–143.

Gobello C, Corrada Y (2002) Noninfectious prostatic diseases in dogs. *Compendium on Continuing Education for the Practising Veterinarian* **24**, 99–107.

Holt PE, White RAS (2000) Prostatic cysts and abscesses in the dog: treatment options. *Veterinary International* **12**, 11–18.

L'Esplattenier HF, Nimwegen SA Van, Sluijs FJ Van *et al.* (2006) Partial prostatectomy using Nd:YAG laser for management of canine prostate carcinoma. *Veterinary Surgery* **35**, 406–411.

Liptak JM, Brutscher SP, Monnet E *et al.* (2004) Transurethral resection in the management of urethral and prostatic neoplasia in 6 dogs. *Veterinary Surgery* **33**, 505–516.

Mullen HS, Matthiesen DT, Scavelli TD (1990) Results of surgery and postoperative complications in 92 dogs treated for prostate abscessation by a multiple Penrose drain technique. *Journal of the American Animal Hospital Association* **26**, 369–379.

Schulz KS, Waldron DR, Smith MM *et al.* (1996) Inadvertent prostatectomy as a complication of cryptorchidectomy in four dogs. *Journal of the American Animal Hospital Association* **32**, 211–214.

Sirinarumitr K, Johnston SD, Root Kustritz MV *et al.* (2001) Effects of finasteride on size of the prostate gland and semen quality in dogs with benign prostatic hypertrophy. *Journal of the American Veterinary Medical Association* **218**, 1275–1280.

Sirinarumitr K, Sirinarumitr T, Johnston SD *et al.* (2002) Finasteride-induced prostatic involution by aptosis in dogs with benign prostatic hypertrophy. *American Journal of Veterinary Research* **63**, 495–498.

Vlasin M, Rauser P, Fichtel T *et al.* (2006) Subtotal intracapsular prostatectomy as a useful treatment for advanced-stage prostatic malignancies. *Journal of Small Animal Practice* **47**, 512–516.

Wasmer ML, Rogers KS (1996) Pharmacologic androgen deprivation. *Compendium on Continuing Education for the Practising Veterinarian* **18**, 267–277.

White RAS, Williams JM (1995) Intracapsular prostatic omentalisation: a new technique for management of prostatic abscesses in dogs. *Veterinary Surgery* **24**, 390–395.

Williams J, Niles J (1999) Prostatic disease in the dog. *In Practice* **21**, 558–575.

Chapter 6: Urinary tract trauma

Anderson RB, Aronson LR, Drobatz KJ *et al.* (2006) Prognostic factors for successful outcome following urethral rupture in dogs and cats. *Journal of the American Animal Hospital Association* **42**, 136–146.

Baines SJ, Rennie S, White RAS (2001) Prepubic urethrostomy: a long-term study in 16 cats. *Veterinary Surgery* **30**, 107–113.

Bernarde A, Viguier E (2004) Transpelvic urethrostomy in 11 cats using an ischial ostectomy. *Veterinary Surgery* **33**, 246–252.

Hamilton MH, Sissener TR, Baines SJ (2006) Traumatic bilateral ureteric rupture in two dogs. *Journal of Small Animal Practice* **47**, 737–740.

Hay CW, Rosin E (1997) Repair of an intrapelvic urethral tear in a bitch caused by iatrogenic trauma. *Veterinary Record* **140**, 48–49.

Moores AP, Bell AMD, Costello M (2002) Urinoma (para-ureteral pseudocyst) as a consequence of trauma in a cat. *Journal of Small Animal Practice* **43**, 213–216.

Nwadike BS, Wilson LP, Stone EA (2000) Use of bilateral temporary nephrostomy catheters for emergency treatment of bilateral ureter transection in a cat. *Journal of the American Veterinary Medical Association* **217**, 1862–1865.

Weisse C, Aronson LR, Drobatz KD (2002) Traumatic rupture of the ureter: 10 cases. *Journal of the American Animal Hospital Association* **38**, 188–192.

Chapter 7: Other causes of haematuria

Agut A, Laredo FG, Belda E *et al.* (2004) Left perinephric abscess associated with nephrolithiasis and bladder calculi in a bitch. *Veterinary Record* **154**, 562–565.

Bolliger C, Walshaw R, Kruger JM *et al.* (2005) Evaluation of the effects of nephrotomy on renal function in clinically normal cats. *American Journal of Veterinary Research* **66**, 1400–1407.

Bryan JN, Henry CJ, Tumquist SE *et al.* (2006) Primary renal neoplasia of dogs. *Journal of Veterinary Internal Medicine* **20**, 1155–1160.

Buffington CAT, Chew DJ, Woodworth BE (1999) Feline interstitial cystitis. *Journal of the American Veterinary Medical Association* **215**, 682–687.

Buffington CAT, Westropp JL, Chew DJ *et al.* (2006) Risk factors associated with clinical signs of lower urinary tract disease in indoor housed cats. *Journal of the American Veterinary Medical Association* **228**, 722–725.

Castellano MC, Idiart JR (2005) Multifocal renal cystadenocarcinoma and nodular dermatofibrosis in dogs. *Compendium on Continuing Education for the Practising Veterinarian* **27**, 846–853.

Chun R, Knapp DW, Widmer WR *et al.* (1996) Cisplatin treatment of transitional cell carcinoma of the urinary bladder in dogs: 18 cases (1982–1993). *Journal of the American Veterinary Medical Association* **209**, 1588–1591.

Cuypers M-LD, Grooters AM, Williams J *et al.* (1997) Renomegally in dogs and cats. Part I. Differential diagnoses. *Compendium on Continuing Education for the Practising Veterinarian* **19**, 1019–1032.

Dobson JM, Samuel S, Milstein H *et al.* (2002) Canine neoplasia in the UK: estimates of incidence rates from a population of insured dogs. *Journal of Small Animal Practice* **43**, 240–246.

Dunning M, Stonehewer J (2002) Urinary tract infections in small animals: pathophysiology and diagnosis. *In Practice* **24**, 418–432.

Dunning M, Stonehewer J (2002) Urinary tract infections in small animals: therapeutic options and management of problem cases. *In Practice* **24**, 518–527.

Eddlestone S, Taboade J, Senior D *et al.* (1999) Renal haemangioma in a dog. *Journal of Small Animal Practice* **40**, 132–135.

Farrell M, Philbey AW, Ramsey I (2006) Ureteral fibroepithelial polyp in a dog. *Journal of Small Animal Practice* **47**, 409–412.

Gasser AM, Bush WW, Smith S *et al.* (2003) Extradural spinal, bone marrow, and renal nephroblastoma. *Journal of the American Animal Hospital Association* **39**, 80–85.

Holt PE, Lucke VM, Pearson H (1987) Idiopathic renal haemorrhage in the dog. *Journal of Small Animal Practice* **28**, 253–263.

Jens B, Bjorling DE (2001) Suture selection for lower urinary tract surgery in small animals. *Compendium on Continuing Education for the Practising Veterinarian* **23**, 524–531.

Kalkstein TS, Kruger JM, Osborne CA (1999) Feline idiopathic lower urinary tract disease. Part II. Potential causes. *Compendium on Continuing Education for the Practising Veterinarian* **21**, 148–155.

Kalkstein TS, Kruger JM, Osborne CA (1999) Feline idiopathic lower urinary tract disease. Part III. Diagnosis. *Compendium on Continuing Education for the Practising Veterinarian* **21**, 387–394, 448.

Kalkstein TS, Kruger JM, Osborne CA (1999) Feline idiopathic lower urinary tract disease. Part IV. Therapeutic options. *Compendium on Continuing Education for the Practising Veterinarian* **21**, 497–509.

King MD, Waldron DR, Barber DL *et al.* (2006) Effect of nephrotomy on renal function and morphology in normal cats. *Veterinary Surgery* **35**, 749–758.

Kirsch JA, Hauptman JG, Walshaw R (2002) A urethropexy technique for surgical treatment of urethral prolapse in the male dog. *Journal of the American Animal Hospital Association* **38**, 381–384.

Knapp DW, Richardson RC, Chan TCK *et al.* (1994) Piroxicam therapy in 34 dogs with transitional cell carcinoma of the urinary bladder. *Journal of Veterinary Internal Medicine* **8**, 273–278.

Knottenbelt C, Chambers G, Gault E *et al.* (2006) The *in vitro* effects of piroxicam on canine cell lines. *Journal of Small Animal Practice* **47**, 14–20.

Knottenbelt C, Mellor D, Nixon C *et al.* (2006) Cohort study of COX-1 and COX-2 expression in canine rectal and bladder tumours. *Journal of Small Animal Practice* **47**, 196–200.

Kyles AE, Hardie EM, Wooden BG *et al.* (2005) Clinical, clinicopathologic, radiographic, and ultrasonographic abnormalities in cats with ureteral calculi: 163 cases (1984–2002). *Journal of the American Veterinary Medical Association* **226**, 932–936.

Kyles AE, Hardie EM, Wooden BG *et al.* (2005) Management and outcome of cats with ureteral calculi: 153 cases (1984–2002). *Journal of the American Veterinary Medical Association* **226**, 937–944.

Mellanby RJ, Chantrey JC, Baines EA *et al.* (2004) Urethral haemangiosarcoma in a Boxer. *Journal of Small Animal Practice* **45**, 154–156.

Moe L, Lum B (1997) Hereditary multifocal cystadenocarcinomas and nodular dermatofibrosis in 51 German shepherd dogs. *Journal of Small Animal Practice* **38**, 498–505.

Phillips BS (1999) Bladder tumors in dogs and cats. *Compendium on Continuing Education for the Practising Veterinarian* **21**, 540–547.

Sale CSH, Skerritt GC, Smith KC (2004) Spinal nephroblastoma in a crossbreed dog. *Journal of Small Animal Practice* **45**, 267–271.

Saridomichelakis MN, Koutinas CK, Souftas V *et al.* (2004) Extensive caudal vena cava thrombosis secondary to unilateral renal tubular cell carcinoma in a dog. *Journal of Small Animal Practice* **45**, 108–112.

Senior DF, Lawrence DT, Gunson C *et al.* (1994) Successful treatment of botryoid rabdomyosarcoma in the bladder of a dog. *Journal of the American Veterinary Medical Association* **29**, 386–390.

Stone EA, Robertson JL, Metcalf MR (2002) The effect of nephrotomy on renal function and morphology in dogs. *Veterinary Surgery* **31**, 391–397.

Westropp JL, Kass PH, Buffington CAT (2006) Evaluation of the effects of stress in cats with idiopathic cystitis. *American Journal of Veterinary Research* **67**, 731–736.

Chapter 8: Urinary incontinence

Aaron A, Eggleton E, Power C *et al.* (1996) Urethral sphincter mechanism incompetence in male dogs: a retrospective analysis of 54 cases. *Veterinary Record* **139**, 542–546.

Arnold S, Jager P, DiBartola SP *et al.* (1989) Treatment of urinary incontinence in dogs by endoscopic injection of Teflon. *Journal of the American Veterinary Medical Association*, **195**, 1369–1374.

Arnold S, Hubler M, Lott-Stolz G *et al.* (1996) Treatment of urinary incontinence in bitches by endoscopic injection of glutaraldehyde cross-linked collagen. *Journal of Small Animal Practice* **37**, 163–168.

Atalan G, Holt PE, Barr FJ (1998) Ultrasonographic assessment of bladder neck mobility in continent bitches and bitches with urinary incontinence attributable to urethral sphincter mechanism incompetence. *American Journal of Veterinary Research* **59**, 673–679.

Bacon NJ, Oni O, White RAS (2002) Treatment of urethral sphincter mechanism incompetence in 11 bitches with a sustained-release formulation of phenylpropanolamine hydrochloride. *Veterinary Record* **151**, 373–376.

Barth A, Reichler IM, Hubler M *et al.* (2005) Evaluation of long-term effects of endoscopic injection of collagen into the urethral submucosa for treatment of urethral sphincter mechanism incompetence in female dogs: 40 cases (1993–2000). *Journal of the American Veterinary Medical Association* **226**, 73–76.

Blavais JG (2005) What to do? *Neurourology and Urodynamics* **24**, 201.

Cannizzo KL, McLoughlin MA, Mattoon JS *et al.* (2003) Evaluation of transurethral cystoscopy and excretory urography for diagnosis of ectopic ureters in female dogs; 25 cases (1992–2000). *Journal of the American Veterinary Medical Association* **223**, 475–481.

Carofiglio F, Hamaide AJ, Farnir F *et al.* (2006) Evaluation of the urodynamic effects of orally administered phenylpropanolamine and ephedrine in female dogs. *American Journal of Veterinary Research* **67**, 723–730.

Chen X, Creed KE (2004) Histochemical and contractile properties of striated muscles of urethra and levator ani of dogs and sheep. *Neurourology and Urodynamics* **23**, 702–708.

Crawford JT, Adams WM (2002) Influence of vestibulovaginal stenosis, pelvic bladder, and recessed vulva on response to treatment for clinical signs of lower urinary tract disease in dogs: 38 cases (1990–1999). *Journal of the American Veterinary Medical Association* **221**, 995–999.

Dean PW, Novotny MJ, O'Brien DP (1989) Prosthetic sphincter for urinary incontinence: results in three cases. *Journal of the American Animal Hospital Association* **25**, 447–454.

Gregory SP, Holt PE (1992) Effect of body position on intravesical pressure in the anaesthetised bitch. *Veterinary Record* **130**, 288–290.

Gregory SP, Parkinson TJ, Holt PE (1992) Urethral conformation and position in relation to urinary incontinence in the bitch. *Veterinary Record* **131**, 167–170.

Gregory SP, Holt PE (1993) Comparison of stressed simultaneous urethral pressure profiles between anesthetized continent and incontinent bitches with urethral sphincter mechanism incompetence. *American Journal of Veterinary Research* **54**, 216–222.

Gregory SP, Holt PE (1994) The immediate effect of colposuspension on resting and stressed urethral pressure profiles in anaesthetized incontinent bitches. *Veterinary Surgery* **23**, 330–340.

Gregory SP, Holt PE, Parkinson TJ *et al.* (1999) Vaginal position and length in the bitch: relationship to spaying and urinary incontinence. *Journal of Small Animal Practice* **40**, 180–184.

Hamaide AJ, Verstegen JP, Snaps FR *et al.* (2005) Influence of the estrous cycle on urodynamic and morphometric measurements of the lower portion of the urogenital tract in dogs. *American Journal of Veterinary Research* **66**, 1075–1083.

Hardie RJ, Schmiedt C, Phillips L *et al.* (2005) Ureteral papilla implantation as a technique for neoureterocystostomy in cats. *Veterinary Surgery* **34**, 393–398.

Holt PE (1983) Urinary incontinence in the dog. *In Practice* **5**, 162–173.

Holt PE (1984) Efficacy of emepronium bromide in the treatment of physiological incontinence in the bitch. *Veterinary Record* **114**, 355–356.

Holt PE (1985) Urinary incontinence in the bitch due to sphincter mechanism incompetence: prevalence in referred dogs and retrospective analysis of sixty cases. *Journal of Small Animal Practice* **26**, 181–190.

Holt PE (1985) Importance of urethral length, bladder neck position and vestibulovaginal stenosis in sphincter mechanism incompetence in the incontinent bitch. *Research in Veterinary Science* **39**, 364–372.

Holt PE (1985) Urinary incontinence in the bitch due to sphincter mechanism incompetence: surgical treatment. *Journal of Small Animal Practice* **26**, 237–246.

Holt PE (1988) 'Simultaneous' urethral pressure profilometry: comparisons between continent and incontinent bitches. *Journal of Small Animal Practice* **29**, 761–769.

Holt PE (1990) Urinary incontinence in dogs and cats. *Veterinary Record* **127**, 347–350.

Holt PE (1990) Long-term evaluation of colposuspension in the treatment of urinary incontinence due to incompetence of the urethral sphincter mechanism in the bitch. *Veterinary Record* **127**, 537–542.

Holt PE (1993) Surgical management of congenital urethral sphincter mechanism incompetence in eight female cats and a bitch. *Veterinary Surgery* **22**, 98–104.

Holt PE (1994) Feline urinary incontinence. In *Kirk's Current Veterinary Therapy XII. Small Animal Practice*. (eds JD Bonagura, RW Kirk) WB Saunders, Philadelphia, pp. 1018–1022.

Holt PE (2000) FECAVA LECTURE. Investigation and therapy of incontinent animals. *European Journal of Companion Animal Practice* **10**, 111–116.

Holt PE, Sayle B (1981) Congenital vestibulo-vaginal stenosis in the bitch. *Journal of Small Animal Practice* **22**, 67–75.

Holt PE, Long SE, Gibbs C (1983) Disorders of urination associated with canine intersexuality. *Journal of Small Animal Practice* **24**, 475–487.

Holt PE, Gibbs C (1992) Congenital urinary incontinence in cats: a review of 19 cases. *Veterinary Record* **130**, 437–442.

Holt PE, Gibbs C, Wathes CM (1990) Simultaneous urethral pressure profilometry using a microtip transducer catheter in the bitch: effects of bitch position and transducer orientation. *Neurourology and Urodynamics* **9**, 281–296.

Holt PE, Gregory SP (1993) Resting urethral pressure profilometry in bitches: artefact or reality? *Compendium on Continuing Education for the Practising Veterinarian* **15**, 1207–1215.

Holt PE, Thrusfield MV (1993) Association in bitches between breed, size, neutering and docking, and acquired urinary incontinence due to incompetence of the urethral sphincter mechanism. *Veterinary Record*, **133**, 177–180.

Holt PE, Hotson Moore A (1995) Canine ureteral ectopia: an analysis of 175 cases and comparison of surgical treatments. *Veterinary Record* **136**, 345–349.

Holt PE, Stone EA (1998) Colposuspension for urinary incontinence. In *Current Techniques in Small Animal Surgery* (4th edn). (ed MJ Bojrab). Williams and Wilkins, Baltimore, pp. 455–459.

Holt PE, Jones A (2000) *In vitro* study of the significance of bladder neck position in incontinent bitches. *Veterinary Record* **146**, 437–439.

Holt PE, Thrusfield MV, Hotson Moore A (2000) Breed predisposition to ureteral ectopia in bitches in the UK. *Veterinary Record* **146**, 561.

Holt PE, Coe RJ, Hotson Moore A (2005) Prostatopexy as a treatment for urethral sphincter mechanism incompetence in male dogs. *Journal of Small Animal Practice* **46**, 567–570.

Kyles AE, Vaden S, Hardie EM *et al.* (1996) Vestibulovaginal stenosis in dogs: 18 cases (1987–1995). *Journal of the American Veterinary Medical Association* **209**, 1889–1893.

Laverty PH, Salisbury SK (2002) Surgical management of true patent urachus in a cat. *Journal of Small Animal Practice* **43**, 227–229.

Lose G, Griffiths D, Hosker G *et al.* (2002) Standardisation of urethral pressure measurement: report from the Standardisation Sub–Committee of the International Continence Society. *Neurourology and Urodynamics* **21**, 258–260.

Mandigers PJJ, Nell T (2001) Treatment of bitches with acquired urinary incontinence with oestriol. *Veterinary Record* **149**, 764–767.

Massat BJ, Gregory CR, Ling GV *et al.* (1993) Cystourethropexy to correct refractory urinary incontinence due to urethral sphincter mechanism incompetence. Preliminary results in ten bitches. *Veterinary Surgery* **22**, 260–268.

McLoughlin MA, Chew DJ (2000) Diagnosis and surgical management of ectopic ureters. *Clinical Techniques in Small Animal Practice* **15**, 17–24.

Mehl ML, Kyles AE, Pollard R *et al.* (2005) Comparison of 3 techniques for ureteroneocystostomy in cats. *Veterinary Surgery* **34**, 114–119.

Michell AR (1984) Ins and outs of bladder function. *Journal of Small Animal Practice* **25**, 237–247.

Muir P, Goldsmid SE, Bellenger CR (1994) Management of urinary incontinence in five bitches with incompetence of the urethral sphincter mechanism by colposuspension and a modified sling urethroplasty. *Veterinary Record* **134**, 38–41.

Nickel RF (1999) Oestriol: pharmacology and effects on lower urinary tract function. *European Society of Veterinary Internal Medicine Newsletter* **9**, 13–15.

Nickel RF, Wiegand U, Van Den Brom WE (1998) Evaluation of a transpelvic sling procedure with and without colposuspension for treatment of femlae dogs with refractory urethral sphincter mechanism incompetence. *Veterinary Surgery* **27**, 94–104.

Nickel RF, Van Den Brom WE, Vink-Noteboom M (1999) Clinical and radiographic findings compared with urodynamic findings in neutered female dogs with refractory urinary incontinence. *Veterinary Record* **145**, 11–15.

Okkens AC, Kooistra HS, Nickel RF (1997) Comparison of long-term effects of ovariectomy versus ovariohysterectomy in bitches. *Journal of Reproduction and Fertility Supplements* **51**, 227–231.

Power SC, Eggleton KE, Aaron AJ et al. (1998) Urethral sphincter mechanism incompetence in the male dog: importance of bladder neck position, proximal urethral length and castration. *Journal of Small Animal Practice* **39**, 69–72.

Rawlings CA, Mahaffey MB, Chernosky AC et al. (2000) Immediate urodynamic and anatomic response to colposuspension in female Beagles. *American Journal of Veterinary Research* **61**, 1353–1357.

Rawlings CA, Barsanti JA, Mahaffey MB et al. (2001) Evaluation of colposuspension for treatment of incontinence in spayed female dogs. *Journal of the American Veterinary Medical Association* **219**, 770–775.

Rawlings CA, Coates CR, Purinton PT et al. (2005) Evaluation of a selective neurectomy model for low urethral pressure incontinence in female dogs. *American Journal of Veterinary Research* **66**, 695–699.

Reichler IM, Hubler M, Jöchle W et al. (2003) The effect of GnRH analogs on urinary incontinence after ablation of the ovaries in dogs. *Theriogenology* **60**, 1207–1216.

Richter KP, Ling GV (1985) Clinical response and urethral pressure profile changes after phenylpropanolamine in dogs with primary sphincter incompetence. *Journal of the American Veterinary Medical Association* **187**, 605–611.

Robinson D, Register TC, Carter LR (1998) The effects of delayed hormone replacement therapy on estrogen receptors of the cynomolgus monkey bladder and vagina. *Neurourology and Urodynamics* **17**, 241–247.

Salomon JF, Cotard JP, Viguier E (2002) Management of urethral sphincter mechanism incompetence in a male dog with laparoscopic-guided deferentopexy. *Journal of Small Animal Practice* **43**, 501–505.

Schäfer W, Abrams P, Liao L et al. (2002) Good urodynamic practices: uroflowmetry, filling cystometry, and pressure-flow studies. *Neurourology and Urodynamics* **21**, 261–274.

Scott L, Leddy M, Bernay F et al. (2002) Evaluation of phenylpropanolamine in the treatment of urethral sphincter mechanism incompetence in the bitch. *Journal of Small Animal Practice* **43**, 493–496.

Spain CV, Scarlett JM, Houpt KA (2004) Long-term risks and benefits of early-age gonadectomy in dogs. *Journal of the American Veterinary Medical Association* **224**, 380–387.

Sutherland-Smith J, Jerram RM, Walker AM et al. (2004) Ectopic ureters and ureteroceles in dogs: presentation, cause and diagnosis. *Compendium on Continuing Education for the Practising Veterinarian* **26**, 303–310.

Sutherland-Smith J, Jerram RM, Walker AM et al. (2004) Ectopic ureters and ureteroceles in dogs: treatment. *Compendium on Continuing Education for the Practising Veterinarian* **26**, 311–316.

Thrusfield MV, Holt PE, Muirhead RH (1998) Acquired urinary incontinence in bitches: its incidence and relationship to neutering practices. *Journal of Small Animal Practice* **39**, 559–566.

Weber UT, Arnold S, Hubler M et al. (1997) Surgical treatment of male dogs with urinary incontinence due to urethral sphincter mechanism incompetence. *Veterinary Surgery* **26**, 51–56.

White RAS, Pomeroy CJ (1989) Phenylpropanolamine: an α-adrenergic agent for the management of urinary incontinence in the bitch associated with urethral sphincter mechanism incompetence. *Veterinary Record* **125**, 478–480.

White RN (2001) Urethropexy for the management of urethral sphincter mechanism incompetence in the bitch. *Journal of Small Animal Practice* **42**, 481–486.

Appendices

Appendix 1 **Drug trade-names**

Phosphate and sodium citrate enemas	Fleet ready-to-use enema (133ml), EC De Witt & Co Ltd; Micralax Micro-Enema, UCB Pharmas Ltd
Frusemide injection	Dimazon 5% solution, Intervet
Water-soluble, iodine-based, positive contrast medium	Omnipaque 300 and 350, GE Healthcare; Urografin '150', Schering
Water-soluble lubricating jelly	K-Y Lubricating Jelly, Johnson and Johnson
Cytospin/cytoslide system	Shandon Cytospin/Cytoslides
Sterile ultrasound gel	Ultra/phonic Conductivity Gel, Pharmaceutical Innovations Inc
Boric acid powder	Boricon Sterile Tube, Medical Wire and Equipment Company Ltd
Glycolide/lactide suture material	Vicryl, Ethicon, Polysorb, Tyco
Polydioxanone suture material	PDS*II, Ethicon
Phenylpropanolamine	Propalin, Vétoquinol, Urilin, Dechra
Oestriol	Incurin, Intervet
Diazepam	Valium, Roche

Appendix 2 **Conversion factors**

Haematology	SI units	Factor	Old units
PCV	l/l	100	%
RBCs	x 10^{12}/l	1	x 10^6/μl
Haemoglobin	g/l	0.1	g/dl
MCHC	g/l	0.1	g/dl
Platelets	x 10^9/l	1	x 10^3/μl
WBCs	x 10^9/l	1	x 10^3/μl
Neutrophils	x 10^9/l	1	x 10^3/μl
Lymphocytes	x 10^9/l	1	x 10^3/μl
Monocytes	x 10^9/l	1	x 10^3/μl
Eosinophils	x 10^9/l	1	x 10^3/μl
Basophils	x 10^9/l	1	x 10^3/μl
Biochemistry			
Albumin	g/l	0.1	g/dl
Globulin	g/l	0.1	g/dl
ALT	u/l	1	u/l
Ammonia	μmol/l	1.3636	μg/dl
Amylase	u/l	1	u/l
AST	u/l	1	u/l
Bile acids	μmol/l	0.41	μg/ml
Calcium	mmol/l	4	mg/dl
Cholesterol	mmol/l	38.61	mg/dl
Triglyceride	mmol/l	88.6	mg/dl
CK	u/l	1	u/l
Creatinine	μmol/l	0.0113	mg/dl
Glucose	mmol/l	18	mg/dl
Phosphorus	mmol/l	3.1	mg/dl
LDH	u/l	1	u/l
Lipase	u/l	1	u/l
Magnesium	mmol/l	1	mEq/l
Potassium	mmol/l	1	mEq/l
ALP	u/l	1	u/l
Sodium	mmol/l	1	mEq/l
Total bilirubin	μmol/l	0.059	mg/dl
Total proteins	g/l	0.1	g/dl
Urea nitrogen	mmol/l	2.8	mg/dl